THE KEANE EDGE

Brian Keane is a qualified personal trainer, sports nutritionist and strength and conditioning coach. He is the bestselling author of *The Fitness Mindset* and has travelled the world as a professional speaker. He also hosts the #1 podcast *The Brian Keane Podcast*. Brian is a former primary school teacher turned fitness entrepreneur. After retiring from the world of professional fitness modelling in 2015, he now does ultra-endurance events all around the world. In April 2018, Brian ran the famous Marathon Des Sables, which entails six self-sufficient back-to-back marathons through the Sahara Desert in Morocco; and in February 2019, he ran 230km through the Arctic Circle in the northernmost tip of Sweden.

THE KEANE EDGE

MASTERING THE MINDSET FOR REAL, LASTING FAT LOSS

Brian Keane

Gill Books

Gill Books
Hume Avenue
Park West
Dublin 12
www.gillbooks.ie

Gill Books is an imprint of M.H. Gill and Co.

978 07171 9137 6

Designed by Síofra Murphy
Print origination by Bartek Janczak
Edited by Susan McKeever
Proofread by Neil Burkey
Indexed by Eileen O'Neill
Nutritional consultation by Fiona McCallion (NutritionbyFiona.com)

Printed by Clays Ltd, Suffolk
This book is typeset in 12 on 18pt Minion Pro.

This book is not intended as a substitute for the medical advice of
a physician. The reader should consult a doctor or mental health
professional if they feel it necessary.

*The paper used in this book comes from the wood pulp of managed
forests. For every tree felled, at least one tree is planted, thereby renewing
natural resources.*

A CIP catalogue record for this book is available from the British
Library.

5 4 3 2 1

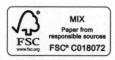

MIX
Paper from
responsible sources
FSC
www.fsc.org
FSC® C018072

This book is dedicated to everyone in my inner circle.
I love you all.

Acknowledgements

There are so many people who I would like to thank for supporting me in the writing of this this book.

Firstly, there are the hundreds of podcast guests who helped to expand my thinking and education around nutrition. Some are mentioned directly in subsequent pages.

I want to thank Sarah, Rachel and all the team at Gill Books. Sarah was instrumental in the shaping of this book, Rachel helped me get it over the finish line and the whole Gill team contributed to bringing it from a concept to a finished product.

I also want to thank my family. My mother, Rita, who has always been my biggest supporter. My father, Gerry, who hardened my mindset to complete things regardless of how I felt. My sister, Karen, who has supported my entire journey from day one. And, of course, my daughter, Holly – who gave my life new meaning in 2015.

My thanks also to Paul Dermody, who helped me hone many of the nutritional philosophies in this book, such as food relationship and not pressing the 'f**k it button'. To my friend and assistant Gary O' Daly, who helped to manage my workload during the writing of this. To Orla O' Flaherty, who challenges me to see things from different perspectives. To Trisha Lewis for introducing me to the team at Gill, the idea of 'resetting' and for being a constant inspiration to me. And to Serena Cabry, for being my rock throughout this entire process. She listened to every one of my rants or monologues when I was stuck writing a particular section.

Thank you all.

Contents

Contents

Introduction

Losing weight is a lot like baking a cake.

Yes, you read that right. I'm starting this 'healthy eating' book talking about baking a cake. As you'll see over the coming chapters, this book is unlike anything you have ever read before. I'm not going to be preaching the fat-burning capabilities of some random food found deep in the Amazon jungle, or selling you on some quick-fix solution that massively reduces your calorie intake by eliminating an entire food group. Nope, you won't get that here. What you *are* going to get in the following pages is a mindset shift.

You're likely going to hear some uncomfortable truths about the sole contributing factor as to why you don't look the way you want to look. I'll give you a clue. When it comes to every single diet or nutritional plan you've followed unsuccessfully over the years, what has been the common denominator? Have you been too restrictive and then pressed the 'f*ck it button' and binged on everything in sight? Possibly. Have you eliminated entire food groups in your desire to lose weight, e.g. six weeks gluten free, no dairy? Yeah, you might have. But none of those is the common denominator. Want to know what is? It's YOU! Yes, you, or more accurately your mindset and how you approach the diet or nutritional plan. But don't worry, we're going to fix that. But first, back to my cake.

Surely cake is off limits if you're trying to lose weight or reduce your body fat? Well, yes and no. Yes in the sense that in Part One of the book you'll see that calories *do* matter and food portion sizes *are* important. Eating a whole cake is unlikely to support your weight-loss goal. Equally though, one slice a few times a week probably has the opposite effect. It gives you the psychological and metabolic boost you need to stick to your nutritional plan over the space of a week, a month or even a year. But that's not why I bring up cake. The reason I bring it up, apart from the fact that cake is delicious, is the baking element.

If you've ever baked a cake (or any other oven treat), you know that you have to follow a recipe. You need to do things in the right order, following a step-by-step process to end up with an appetising baked good. But you also need the ingredient list. Forget the flour and you have a pile of mush, forget the sugar and it tastes horrible, forget the eggs and it doesn't stick together – you get the idea. Developing the Keane Edge is exactly the same. To lose weight, you need the recipe, and you need to follow a step-by-step process. In Part One, we'll go through that: how calories work, what you need to know about macros – the foods that make up your calories – and food choices and the order of priority or 'fat-loss pyramid of prioritisation' that comes alongside them.

At this point, you might be thinking, 'Oh God, not another diet book on clean eating,' or 'To lose weight, consume fewer calories – been there, done that' – oh no my friend, that's just the start of it. Similar to baking a cake, you can know exactly how to make it but it still might taste like crap if you don't know what ingredients to use. Which brings me on to the meat and potatoes (pardon the pun) of this book – the ingredients, aka your mindset tools.

The educational side of the weight-loss process is broken down into everything from calories, macros and food choices to using the correct metrics to track your progress. Randomly following dietary advice without context or knowledge is a recipe for misery. You might hit your weight-loss goal, but you might not. You always want to be able to replicate what you do. For instance, If you lost 4 kilos to look your absolute best for a wedding or other event, you want to be able to replicate that any time you need to in the future. I only use the word 'diet' as an adjective. It's a skill you acquire to use when you need it. You diet to slim down for a date in the future. And unless you are morbidly obese or seriously overweight and you've been dieting for more than a year with no result, you are doing it wrong! Over the course of our journey together, you will acquire the dieting skill but our primary focus will be on the nutrition side of things. That means finding a plan that is specific to your goal and then approaching it the right way. The ingredients come next and the first one on that list is discipline.

THE DISCIPLINE INGREDIENT

When I say 'discipline', I'm not talking about gruelling workout sessions in a gym, or even avoiding your favourite foods to hit a weight-loss target. Far from it. What I mean by discipline is building habits that support your end goal, so that you don't feel like you're on a 'diet'.

Being disciplined is about understanding how your daily actions and behaviours determine how well you do on your weight-loss journey. If you tell me how you eat every day, I'll tell you how much weight you'll lose or how you'll look in a year. I'm also going to break down the myth of motivation and the misconception that there are 'motivated people' out there. Spoiler alert, there's no such thing as 'motivated people' – there are *disciplined* people: individuals with good daily habits or people who have educated themselves and conditioned their mindset to find a nutritional plan that works for them. We can remove that unsupportive belief system of discipline here and now because it's nonsense and only serves as an obstacle to the correct mindset. More on this later. So if discipline is one of our ingredients, what else is there? I'm glad you asked.

THE FAILURE INGREDIENT

Failure is next on the list. Yes, failure is an important ingredient on your journey. But wait, how is failure helpful? Surely that's a bad thing, right? Nope. Failure is one of the most important ingredients on your weight-loss journey because failure isn't final: failure is feedback! Feedback on what hasn't worked in the past. Feedback on how you avoid self-sabotage in the future. In this section, we'll talk about the concept of 'pressing the f*ck it button'. You all know what I'm talking about; you've eaten poorly all day Saturday and then had a big fry up on Sunday morning, so you say, 'F*ck it, I'll start back on my plan tomorrow.' Yeah, you know the button. If it's overused, or worse, worn out, we'll figure out why and put a plan in place around it. Failure also gives us the tool of 'resetting', where you don't let one bad meal turn into two or a bad weekend turn into a bad week. We 'reset' after a potential slip and we get right back on plan. That's failure as feedback and that brings me on to the final ingredient in this recipe: the mindset tools.

THE MINDSET INGREDIENT

This book is ultimately a tool book, and your mindset tools are the most important ones. We'll go through philosophies such as getting your ladder up against the right wall, or in other words, finding the plan that's in alignment with your goals, one that includes foods you enjoy and one that you can stick to. We'll also go over the 0–1 principle on why the start of any new diet is the hardest part, even though it's usually when you're at your most motivated (and why that's normally the problem).

We will go deep on the problem with waiting for Monday if you're feeling motivated on Friday, and the unsupportive behaviour of having a 'last supper' – a ritual that involves bingeing on your favourite foods because you start a diet tomorrow. We'll also go deep on your 'why'. Why do you want to lose weight? Why do you want to reduce your body fat? Why do you want to look a certain way? Knowing why you're doing it can be the difference between success and failure on a dietary plan.

You will come to see that it's not the diet that's the issue: it's your mindset towards it that's been the problem all along. The honest truth is that most diets work if you stick to them. But why can't you stick to your diet? Is it unsustainable? Does it eliminate your favourite foods? Do you feel rubbish on it – low energy, crap sleep, poor sex drive? We'll uncover those tangibles and intangibles as we dive deeper into the book, but for now, realise that this book works with any diet. Although the final part will give you a nutritional plan to follow and some recipes with high-quality, nutrient-dense meals, truthfully any plan will work if you stick to it. What tool do you need to help you with this job? Are you self-sabotaging? Cool, read that section and use the tools in there to help you. Do you lack motivation or have bad dietary habits? Great, check out that chapter and pull out the tools you need.

My mission with this book is to make you realise that outside of some fundamental educational principles that everybody on a weight-loss journey should know – such as basic calorie intake – it's not the diet per se that determines your weight loss success: it's your mindset towards it that matters. Thinking that the diet is the problem – or what I call 'the diet mindset' – is not only flawed, it's broken and downright wrong. And it's time to upgrade your thinking. You can leave that 'diet mindset' at the door. Now we're moving to the next level. The level that gets you exactly where you need to be and keeps you there until your goals change. Now we're talking about the Keane Edge.

HOW TO READ THIS BOOK

Part One of this book is for absolute beginners. If this is the first book on nutrition that you've ever picked up and are confused or don't fully understand calories, macros or how food choices affect your body composition, then I recommend reading Part One in its entirety. If you are already familiar with foundational nutritional principles such as calories and macros, you can skip to the end of Part One, where I've recapped the main takeaways, and then jump into Part Two, which talks about developing the mindset around nutrition. Part Three deals with nutrition itself and training, while Part Four looks at the pivotal but often-misunderstood area of fat loss: sleep and stress.

The book's final part gives you 'The Plan'. It's not the un-sustainable kind of 'one and done' formula you may have come across in other diet books; I'm interested in mindset, nutrition and how to efficiently lose weight or reduce body fat over time. That being said, the plan will help you get started if you're feeling motivated right now.

Part One

The Bear

Part One
The Basics

Calories 101

One of the biggest problems with most diet books is that they don't address the most fundamental thing when it comes to fat loss: the basic understanding of calories. Put simply, the amount of energy contained in an item of food or drink is measured in calories. When we eat and drink more calories than we use, our bodies store the excess as body fat. If this continues, one tends to put on weight over time. It's not unlike a bank balance. If you earn €2,000 per month but spend €2,100 every month, you're going to be broke soon.

Calories work in a similar manner. If your maintenance requires 2,000kcal and you consistently eat 2,100kcal, you're going to gain fat over time. It really is that simple and straightforward. As you'll see later, the types of calories you eat or, more accurately, the macro split or food choices you make, will affect how you look, how you feel and your overall body composition. For now, though, the takeaway message before we continue is that too many calories = weight gain.

HOW MANY CALORIES DO I ACTUALLY NEED?

Since too many calories equals weight gain, it begs the obvious follow-up question: how many calories do I actually need? Generally, the average man needs around 2,500kcal a day to maintain a healthy body weight, and for an average woman, that figure is around 2,000kcal a day. However, these are just ballpark numbers, as individual needs, current goals, activity level and genetics all contribute to how many calories one should be consuming each day.

I'm going to make the assumption that since you're reading a nutrition book, your primary goal is weight or fat loss. I make this assumption because building lean muscle tissue or improving athletic performance normally require a different protocol for calorie calculation; if you have secondary goals outside of fat loss, it's worth factoring them into your overall calorie intake. For example, if you want to lose fat but also build lean muscle tissue or tone up, you might need to keep your calorie intake slightly higher than someone who is solely focused on weight loss.

There are several ways to test and track how many calories you are consuming, and the keyword here is 'test'. A total daily energy expenditure (TDEE) calculator can be extremely useful for addressing the number of calories one needs to consume each day in order to lose weight, but it still needs to be tested. For those unfamiliar with a TDEE calculator, it provides an estimate of how many calories you burn per day, taking exercise into account. It is calculated by first figuring out your basal metabolic rate and then multiplying that value by an activity multiplier. Simply put, it tells you how many calories you need to eat each day, based on your lifestyle, in order to lose fat.

At the end of the day, though, calorie calculators are machine based, and you're not a machine. You're a human being, which means that the way your body is physically responding is a better indicator of progress than any calorie calculator you can find either online or offline. However, these calculators do give you a good starting point; just don't become too obsessed with the number.

I mention this because I've worked in the past with people who are obsessed with their calorie intake. They look at the number on the calculator and track every morsel of food that they put into their mouth. From my experience, the understanding of basic calories is essential, but putting all your energy, effort and self-worth into the numbers is a recipe for misery. I advise using a TDEE calculator to start tracking your calories for a couple of weeks, to get a basic understanding of how many calories you are actually eating every day. After that, it's up to you whether you wish to continue tracking your intake rigorously or take a more lenient approach, such as gauging by eye the amount you are consuming.

THE ONE THING FOR FAT LOSS

After you've calculated your TDEE, you need to get into a calorie deficit. Let's say your individual TDEE number shows up as 1,800kcal per day. This means that any number above this is a calorie *surplus*, which can potentially lead to fat gain. Conversely, any number below this is a calorie *deficit*, which can potentially lead to fat loss. I generally recommend testing your minimum effective dose (MED), which in this scenario means that you focus on consuming 1,700kcal every day, which means a deficit of 100kcal per day. Test this out for 10–14 days, see if your body fat has reduced (discussed below), and then based on that feedback, adjust or maintain your consumption accordingly.

Of course, if you want more drastic results, you go into a more drastic deficit, but as Part Two of this book will explore, make sure you can stick to that deficit. Yes, eating 700kcal every day will give you a 1,000kcal per day deficit, and the logic can be that if I multiply the size of my deficit, I'll multiply results. I'm afraid that's just not the case when it comes to losing body fat. On top of certain hormonal disruptions that occur with severely reducing calories in general populations, adherence can suffer dramatically in these kinds of plans. Things like your mood and energy levels can also plummet. Personally, I very rarely see the need to go for more than 300–500kcal deficit (depending on the TDEE number, of course). Now you test it.

If your body fat isn't decreasing, you need to either decrease your number of calories further or you need to move more (i.e. burn more calories). On the other hand, if you're happy with your progress, just keep doing what you're doing. Now for the most important thing. Make sure you are tracking the correct metric! In other words, make sure you are losing body fat. Why didn't I say 'make sure you are losing weight' here? It's simple. Losing weight and losing body fat are not the same thing.

Losing weight is reducing numbers on a scale. The scale is the metric; it's a unit of measurement. When you step on a scale and it says 50kg, it means you weigh 50kg. If you step on a scale that says 45kg six weeks later, it means you now weigh 45kg. You have lost 5kg of weight. But this may not be 5kg of fat. You may have lost muscle, water weight or even stored glycogen from the carbohydrates you eat, so unless you're severely overweight to begin with, the scales won't really tell you how much body fat you've lost. Having said that, if you *are* clinically overweight or obese, then the scale is a good starting point for tracking your progress. I'm also not saying that you need to throw away your weighing scale, as it can still be a useful method to track progress – just make sure it's not the only way you're tracking your progress.

Although they are different, for the purposes of keeping it simple and using the language you are most familiar with, I will use both 'weight loss' and 'fat loss' interchangeably from here until the end of the book; but be aware that they do not mean the same thing.

IS YOUR BODY FAT DROPPING?

Once you have calculated your TDEE and tracked your calorie consumption for a couple of weeks, it's now time to test if your body fat is decreasing. Although there are many ways to track body fat – from 3D body scanners to hydrostatic weighting (where you get weighed under water) – when it comes to testing body fat reduction, there are four methods that I generally recommend. I'll start with the two that have a higher level of accuracy but are my least favourite of the four.

1. Skinfold calipers

Skinfold calipers measure the thickness of your subcutaneous fat (the fat underneath the skin) at certain locations in the body.

- **Pro:** Skinfold calipers are affordable, portable and measurements can be taken quickly.
- **Con:** The method requires practice and basic knowledge of anatomy. Also, for obvious reasons, some people don't enjoy getting their fat pinched.

2. Dual-energy X-ray absorptiometry (DXA) scan

For some, this is regarded as one of the best, most accurate methods for tracking body fat, but as you'll see, it's not the most readily available method and can be quite costly.

- **Pro:** This method provides accurate and detailed information, including a breakdown of different body regions and bone density readings.
- **Con:** DXAs are often unavailable to the general public, are expensive when available, and deliver a very small amount of radiation.

The two options mentioned above tend to work well for professionals, but what about the person who just wants to look better and check if their fat is reducing or not? This brings me to my two personal favourite ways of tracking body fat. Although neither is technically as accurate as the examples provided above, they are considerably easier to do and cost nothing!

3. Photos

Yes, straightforward and simple. From the first day of my 1:1 personal training journey to now, when I work as an online coach, I always get clients to track their progress from photos. Why? Because the old adage 'a picture is worth a thousand words' holds true when it comes to checking whether body fat is reducing. One of the major problems with losing body fat is that we tend not to see our own progress from day to day (or even week to week in some cases), but as with clothing – which I'll get to next – photos don't lie.

If you're maintaining a calorie deficit, you should see a decrease in your body fat as the days and weeks go by. You might not see it in your most stubborn areas: your bum, your stomach, your hips or lower back and so on, but it will be apparent elsewhere: your arms, your chest and your legs. We'll come back to stubborn body fat later. For now, photos are a great way to track if your body fat is reducing or not.

- **Pro:** Photos are an inexpensive way to track your body fat. They are also very accurate when it comes to body composition, as the visual representation can make progress (or the lack thereof) easy to see.

- **Con:** There isn't a tangible number to work with in the case of photos, unlike the calipers above, and progress can be subjective. So, if you don't have a coach or trainer to look over the photos, it can be difficult to notice progress over shorter periods of time.

My recommendations for taking photos

- Take three photos: one from the front, one from the back and one from the side.

- Wear clothing that shows your body. For females, I recommend a sports bra and underwear or shorts. For males, I recommend underwear or shorts. Remember these photos are for you to track your own progress, and you don't need to share them with anyone. Just make sure all your major body parts are clearly visible.

- Keep the conditions the same every week. Take the photos before you have eaten or drunk anything, in the same room and under the same lighting.

- Have a designated day to take your photos, such as every Friday morning when you wake up.

4. Clothing fit

Again, similar to the option of photos discussed above, how your clothes fit can be a great indicator of progress. If you've dropped a dress size or a trouser size or two, you know your body fat is reducing. One of the reframes I give my clients who are obsessed with the numbers on a scale is asking them about the size of their clothes.

To this day, I've never seen a dress or t-shirt that says, 'You can wear me if you weigh 45kg or 80kg'. Clothing comes in sizes: 16, 14, 12; small, medium, large; 36cm, 34cm, 32cm and so on. If you currently wear a size 16 or 36-cm trousers and, in six weeks, have dropped to a size 14 or 34cm in the waist, there's a good chance you've lost body fat.

- **Pro:** This is a very easy way to track progress. If your old clothes are starting to feel loose on you, it's likely your body fat is reducing.
- **Con:** Although clothing sizes give you a tangible number, sometimes the accuracy of the progress can be misleading.

For example, if you have eliminated certain foods that caused bloating and dropped a pants size as a result, this can skew the results.

CALORIE TRACKING – MAKING IT A HABIT

When it comes to calorie tracking, there are two methodologies that most coaches apply: one is the lenient approach of tracking everything for a week or 10 days and then doing it by eye after that; the other is tracking every morsel of food or drink you consume to further increase your chances of hitting your body composition goal. So which one is better? The answer is neither and, paradoxically, both.

Calorie tracking is like a tool, but similar to any tool, it works great for certain jobs and is terrible for others. Take a hammer, for example. A hammer is a fantastic tool for banging in a nail, however it is not so good if you have a handful of screws. In that instance, a screwdriver is a better tool. I'll go one step further with this analogy, as calorie tracking can be a fantastic tool to support your weight-loss goal in one scenario, but can lead to disordered eating in another.

Using it to identify how many daily calories you are currently eating can go a long way in helping you to lose weight. Equally however, if you have a poor relationship with food, tracking everything you eat can strain or damage that relationship further; so your starting point is important. We will discuss food relationship later on in the book. For now, just think of tracking calories, like the hammer I mentioned above. Remember, you can use it to hammer in the nail, or you can hit yourself in the face with it. It is not the tool that is the problem, it is how you are using it. Here are my top four ways to avoid 'hammer in the face' syndrome that comes with calorie tracking.

Mistakes to avoid and how to track calories correctly

1. **Track everything you eat.** This includes *all* food, drinks and snacks – if it has calories in it, it gets tracked.

2. **Be disciplined and do not fool yourself.** Later in the book, you will see the Seven Deadly Diet Sins and the importance of not lying to yourself about what you are eating. I had a client several years ago who was 14 kilos overweight. She had been dieting on and off for nearly 10 years and was finally at a place where she thought she was making good food choices but still could not lose any weight; so I got her to do me a food diary for the week. She came back to me with a food log that consisted of salad, chicken and two biscuits at lunchtime. This amounted to under 1,000kcal a day. Knowing that something was not adding up, I got her to forensically track every single thing she put into her mouth for the next seven days – and lo and behold, it turned out she was eating closer to 3,000 calories per day. She was indeed having salad at lunchtime, but the dressing that came with it was 600kcal (which she did not include in the log). She was having a good few biscuits, not just the two she claimed; she admitted that she was too embarrassed to tell me this. She was also picking and snacking on nuts and fruits throughout the day. Again, not necessarily 'bad' or unsupportive food choices, but all those calories added up, and she was completely unaware of most of it.

Tracking her calories removed the subjectivity, and all that was left were the facts – the actual calories she was eating every day. After that, it was relatively straightforward to address. We switched the salad dressing, reduced the snacking between meals and even left her with several biscuits every day. She went into a calorie deficit diet plan, and the weight started to fall off. This is just an example of calorie tracking as a tool and how failure can be feedback. The food log did not work, so we went to Plan B. The real success secret is to remove emotion from the actual calorie tracking. You are not trying to fool your coach, me or even yourself. Just use it to get the actual facts of how many calories per day you are eating. If you want to keep eating that way, great, but at least now you understand why you are not reducing body fat.

3. **Find an easy-to-use app.** There is genius in simplicity when it comes to fitness or nutrition apps. Personally, I like MyFitnessPal as a calorie-tracking app, but feel free to search around for one that you find simple to operate. Understand app limitations – calorie-tracking apps are great, but they are not perfect. There can be calorie or brand discrepancies among food labels, so there is always going to be slight chance of error when tracking.[1] For the most part though, they are generally accurate.

4. **Do not get hooked on it.** Unless you are a competitive bodybuilder or a catwalk model, tracking every morsel of food that enters your mouth just is not a very sustainable approach over the long term. Later in the book, I will talk about 'dieting as a skill', and calorie tracking is in the same bracket. If you have a wedding or particular date that you

want to look your very best for, then follow the 'what gets measured gets managed' philosophy and track everything you eat until you hit your goal. Then for the rest of the year, just do it by eye. As we dive deeper into the book, you will see why this is the best approach going forward and knocks you out of the dreaded 'dieting mindset' that is so easy to fall into.

PORTION SIZE AND THE 'RIGHT' CALORIES

Portion size can be the thing the sets people back on their journey, so I want to address it here. Outside of times when you're working towards a special occasion, just keep an eye on your portion size – the amount of food on your plate. If your jeans are starting to feel tighter as the weeks go by, reduce back the portion sizes in your meals slightly.

Let's go into a bit more detail about the calories in the food you eat. Every type of food has calories. A calorie or a kilocalorie (kcal), as we normally refer to it, is a unit of energy. When you hear something contains 100 calories, it is a way of describing how much energy your body could get from eating or drinking it. How calories work when it comes to fat loss or fat gain is pretty straightforward. If you eat too many (calorie surplus), you have taken in too much energy, which your body now stores as excess fat. If you eat too few calories (calorie deficit), your body now has to use stored fat for energy. That is that in a nutshell.

However, when it comes to calories, there are two dominating schools of thought: one says that a calorie is a calorie regardless of where it comes from, and the other that not all calories are created equal, i.e. 100kcal from protein and 100kcal from carbohydrates are absorbed differently by the body.

Like most things, when it comes to nutrition, the truth is somewhere in the middle. True, your body sees calories as just units of energy; so, if you eat 100kcal worth of protein, 100kcal of fat or 100kcal worth of carbohydrate, your body just sees that as 100kcal. In so far as fat loss is considered, this is true. To give you an extreme example, technically, as long as you were in a caloric deficit plan, you could eat only chocolate bars and pizza and still lose weight. Of course, in this figurative scenario, which I do not recommend, the intangible nature of your fat loss would be a cause for concern. Eating this way would lead to low energy levels, poor sex drive and substandard sleep quality, all of which would make the process significantly more difficult to adhere to. Not to mention, your actual body composition would not look as good compared to somebody on a similar calorie plan whose protein requirements and exercise needs were being met.

But just so you are aware, 99 out of 100 people will still reduce fat with this poor-quality diet. How long they'd be able to stick to it with all the intangible negatives mentioned above is another question entirely, but it illustrates the important role calorie intake plays. The other 1 of 100 I'll get to later in this section. Why do I bring this up? Two reasons. One is to show you the importance of calorie intake. You can eat a very low-nutrient albeit low-calorie diet and still lose fat, which I obviously do not recommend. Equally, you can eat a diet entirely comprised of chicken, broccoli and rice, but if it puts you into a calorie surplus, your body fat is still likely to go up. As you will see in later chapters, I am a massive proponent of building a nutritional plan that is 80 per cent grounded in nutrient-dense, high-quality food – lots of fruits and vegetables, complex carbohydrates, healthy fats, complete protein foods and 20 per cent made up of your favourite foods that help you stay on plan – chocolate, crisps, soda, etc.

Although there are more important things to consider with the thesis of this book, the takeaway from calorie tracking and portion sizes is be aware of them; understand the role they play, but do not overthink or overcomplicate it.

STUBBORN BODY FAT

You know it, I know it, we all know it. It's that dreaded area where stubborn body fat accumulates. Most people have an area of stubborn fat in their body, an area that has resisted all efforts of weight loss through diet and exercise and just won't go away. This stubborn fat is usually the fat just under our skin, which you can pinch. It is the subcutaneous fat, as opposed to the visceral fat that wraps around internal organs such as your liver and pancreas. Stubborn fat is incredibly frustrating, especially when you eat healthily and exercise regularly but still can't seem to affect it in any way.

The reality is that your area of stubborn body fat, as the name suggests, is going to be the last place where your body fat reduces. Over the years, I've worked with hundreds of clients who have struggled with their stubborn fat, and their results have normally come from asking two simple questions and understanding the cognitive bias that underpins human behaviour when it comes to fat reduction.

Cognitive bias is defined as a 'systemic error in thinking that occurs when people are processing and interpreting information in the world around them and affects the decisions and judgements that they make'.[2] The two questions that can regularly spark a breakthrough in this area are:

1. Is your body fat reducing everywhere else?
2. Are you focusing on the area that you least like about yourself?

The action bias

If your body fat is reducing everywhere else, then you need to learn one thing: patience, the most unsexy yet the most beneficial skill to acquire when it comes to reducing stubborn body fat. Yes, somebody, somewhere will promise you the 'quick fix', the magic pills in the form of supplements or the remarkable formula or strategy that's being peddled by some online health or fitness guru, but the reality is that all they do is make you feel like you're doing something and it normally comes at a considerable cost. The action bias, where we tend to think that value can only be realised through action, is a catch-22 of human behaviour. It can be a very useful approach in a lot of cases, for example by reading an educational book on nutrition, getting up to do a workout or preparing your meals in advance. But the action bias that makes you want to jump on to the next diet, supplement or formula that promises extreme results in a very unrealistic time period is totally unsupportive. Understanding the difference can form your foundation to cultivating patience and the mindset of 'If it sounds too good to be true, it probably is'. We will get to that in Part Two of this book. If you are reducing fat from all over your body, except for your stubborn areas, then you must keep doing what you're doing. Eventually, you will tap into those stubborn fat stores too.

The negativity bias

This brings me to the second most frequent observation when it comes to your mindset towards stubborn body fat: the question, 'Is the negativity bias drawing your attention to the area you least like about yourself?' Alongside the action bias mentioned above, the negativity bias can also set you up for failure. The negativity bias is our tendency to not only register negative stimuli more readily but to also dwell on these events. Also known as positive-negative asymmetry, this negativity bias means that we feel the sting of a rebuke more powerfully than we do the joy of praise. In the context of your body composition, it means that you disproportionately focus on the areas you're unhappy with more than the areas that are actually improving.

I've worked with many clients who struggle to see how well they're actually progressing because they focus too much on the part of their body that they are not currently happy with. Their clothes might be looser, their body fat lower in their legs, bum, back and arms, but they can't seem to shift the fat from the front of their stomach and that's all they can focus on. In reality, what you focus on is what will occupy most space in your mind, so start focusing on the positive elements of your body, especially if you're progressing in the right direction, and trust the process. As I have mentioned above, if your body fat is reducing everywhere else, it's only a matter of time before your stubborn area reduces too.

Does exercise choice affect stubborn body fat?

Yes and no. No in the sense that you can't spot-reduce fat: you can't do crunches just to lose stubborn fat around your stomach.

However, exercise increases the number of calories burnt, and with a calorie deficit, you will lose fat from all over your body, not just the part you are working on. So, while crunches are good for building strength and working out the muscles around the abdomen, they won't burn off stubborn fat in that area.

That being said, some people will lose fat at a faster rate from some parts of their bodies compared to others, and where the fat melts off first varies from one person to another and, until human physiology changes, there's not a lot that can be done about that.

Are hormones to blame?

Again, yes and no. Hormones can be a little bit of a chicken-and-egg scenario. Is body fat high because hormones aren't balanced or are hormones unbalanced because the body fat is high? It's a never-ending question for fitness professionals, and from my experience, truth be told, it doesn't really matter. The reason I even mention hormones here is that a lot of people have the misconception that their hormones are to blame.

In my online programme, I have worked with many people who come to me with 'I think my hormones are all over the place, and that's why I can't lose weight' or some variation of this sentence. In 99.9 per cent of the cases, those people were not in a calorie deficit. Either they weren't tracking their calorie intake in general or they miscalculated their requirements based on their activity levels, but as soon as we put them into a calorie deficit, the fat started melting away.

Occasionally, somebody *will* come to me with a hormonal disruption, sometimes a result of lifestyle choices but, in most cases, due to extreme dietary restrictions adopted in an effort to lose weight. For these people, fat, and stubborn fat in particular, continues to cling to areas of the body even when they are in a calorie deficit. In women, fat primarily stored in the lower body is often due to the impact of the hormone oestrogen. Higher levels of cortisol (the stress hormone) can also cause the body to hang on to fat. The bottom line is, if your waistline is getting bigger while you're in a calorie deficit and exercising regularly, hormones *could* be to blame. I recommend seeking professional help with a hormone specialist in this scenario.

The hormones worth knowing about

When it comes to weight loss or fat reduction, there are two hormones, ghrelin and leptin, that are especially important to understand. Knowing about them can be useful in learning why you feel the way you do on certain diets, and why certain diets tend to be more successful or have a higher rate of success than others. Conversely, it could explain why some overly restrictive nutritional strategies are doomed to failure from the get-go, purely from a hormonal and physiological standpoint. For example, most bar, shake or juice diets tend to fall into this bracket.

Ghrelin

Ghrelin, also known as the 'hunger hormone', is produced in the stomach, and its function is to tell the brain that the body has to be fed. Ghrelin is generally mediated by your circadian rhythm – the sleep and wake cycle – so maintaining relatively regular eating times each day is a good strategy for managing hunger levels. We'll come back to circadian rhythms in the sleep chapter. Ghrelin can be disrupted by poor sleep or increased during calorie restriction. One of the reasons why certain diets that overly restrict calorie intake are so difficult to stick to is the downregulation in this hormone. Being hungry all the time is a recipe for failure with any nutritional plan. Short-term or acute hunger is fine, as your body becomes accustomed to a reduced caloric intake, but chronic or long-term hunger normally means a nutrient deficiency in the foods you're eating, or that your quantity of food is just too low.

How to manage ghrelin levels:
- Focus on getting high-quality sleep each night.
- Maintain regular eating times every day.
- Don't overly restrict calories for long periods of time. This is not to be confused with being in a caloric deficit for long periods of time. If you are extremely overweight or obese, you can maintain a calorie deficit for months and potentially years on end, as your body has stored fat to use for fuel. By 'overly restrict', I mean eating a calorie intake that is dramatically below your maintenance calorie number, e.g. your maintenance calories are 2,500 but you eat 1,000kcal every day.

Leptin

Leptin is part of a group of hormones called adipokines, which are exclusively released from fat cells. Leptin sends signals to your brain to reduce hunger, decrease appetite/cravings and increase spontaneous activity (your non-exercise activity thermogenesis – NEAT), i.e. fidgeting, walking around more, etc. If ghrelin is considered the 'hunger hormone', leptin can be called the 'full hormone'. Leptin is considered to be a homeostatic driver designed to help you maintain a certain weight because as your fat cells store more fatty acids, leptin secretion increases and your appetite goes down. Likewise, as your fat cells are emptied due to reductions in body fat, leptin levels increase along with appetite. To achieve long-term weight loss, it's important not to make any drastic dietary changes, which can lead to an increase in ghrelin and a decrease in leptin, causing hunger, increased appetite, reduced motivation to exercise and a decreased number of calories burnt at rest.

Now let's get into the *real* thing that determines your dietary success: your mindset!

Take Action

1. Calculate your TDEE.
2. Download a calorie tracker on your phone.

PART ONE TAKEAWAYS

- Your maintenance calories constitute the number of calories you need to stay the same weight.
- A calorie surplus is any number above your maintenance calories (which can lead to weight gain).
- A calorie deficit is any number below your maintenance calories (which can lead to weight loss).
- A calorie deficit is the *one thing* you need to do to lower body fat.
- A total daily energy expenditure (TDEE) calculator is a good way to figure out how many calories you need to eat each day in order to reduce body fat.
- Weight loss is lowering numbers on a scale. Losing body fat is reducing the amount of fat on your body.
- Skinfold calipers and DXA scanners are good professional tools for tracking body fat.
- Photos and the fit of your clothes are inexpensive and easier ways to track your body fat.
- Tracking calories and understanding portion control is important, but don't overthink or overcomplicate it.
- Losing stubborn body fat is down to patience and potentially rewiring your mindset around the area on which you focus your attention.
- You may have an issue with hormones and weight loss, but it's more likely that you're not in a calorie deficit if the weight is not reducing.
- Ghrelin is your 'hunger' hormone.
- Leptin is your 'full' hormone.

Part Two
The Mindset

Why things have gone wrong in the past

There is a story that I think anyone interested in human psychology ought to know. It comes in many forms, but here's the version given to me by one of my family members.

A policeman sees a drunk man searching for something under a streetlight and asks the drunk what he has lost. He tells the policeman he lost his keys and they both look under the streetlight together. After a few minutes, the policeman asks him if he is sure he lost them there, and the drunk replies, 'No, I lost them in the park.' The policeman then asks him why he is searching for the keys there, and the drunk replies, 'This is where the light is.'

That's exactly how weight loss can be. You are looking for the right thing: a leaner physique, a body that makes you feel more confident, or that feeling of sexiness both in and out of your clothes. But in a similar manner as the drunk above, you're looking for it in the wrong place. If you've ever jumped on to the next 'new' diet or have done a bar, shake or 'detox' plan, it's the dietary equivalent of the drunk looking for his keys in the wrong location. Thankfully, this book is going to change all that.

Let's look at what is probably the biggest misconception in all of nutrition: that diets work for weight loss. It is what I like to call 'The Diet Paradox'.

THE DIET PARADOX

In simple terms, a paradox is something you believe to be true when in fact the opposite is normally the case. In this context, I'm talking about diets. For most of your adult life, you've probably believed that dieting is the best way to lose weight or, even worse, the only way to do so. I'm going to explain why that just isn't true. Diets, by their very nature, are difficult. Before we continue, I must clarify that the word 'diet' is not to be confused with nutrition or, as I will refer to it for the rest of the section, 'nutritional plan'. Nutrition is the way you eat. It's generally considered to be a lifestyle. A 'diet' is something you follow until you hit some set target, such as losing 10 kilos, dropping two dress sizes, toning up more and so on, after which you go back to your 'normal' way of eating.

Normally, when we decide to go on a diet, there is some external factor that is influencing our behaviour and mindset – an upcoming event or even the desire to look good naked in front of a new or current romantic partner. The motivation may also be more extreme: a health scare or a nasty comment or jibe from a friend or a loved one – in some cases, even a random stranger

– but it's still something external that has inwardly manifested itself into us deciding that we need to make a change.

Now, before I continue, just to play the devil's advocate, dieting can be a very useful skill. And I use the word 'skill' in the most literal sense. A skill is something you acquire over time and use when you have to. If you learn the skill of boxing, it can be useful if someone tries to mug you down a back alley. Dieting is similar. In some situations, understanding how to 'diet' can be a useful tool in your arsenal, and if you're a competitive bodybuilder, bikini competitor or a fitness model, it's a basic skill to learn. But I'm going to now argue why this diet mentality is all wrong if you're seeking to lose weight, reduce body fat or just look and feel your best.

If you've been dieting half your adult life, you're doing it wrong!

Over the years, I've worked with countless clients whose primary goal is weight loss or fat reduction. As mentioned in Part One of this book, these two aims are not to be confused. An orange and a lemon are both fruits, but they're different. Weight loss and fat reduction are both fitness goals, but they're different. Remember: losing weight is reducing numbers on a scale; losing body fat is reducing the amount of fat in your body.

When I worked as a 1:1 personal trainer, a common story I would hear from potential clients related to how they had been 'on and off' diets for the past five, ten or even fifteen years. In 2014, I was working with a woman who was about 11 kilos overweight. When she came to me, she was 30 years of age and had been dieting on and off since she was 20. I asked her why she had reached out to me about coaching. She replied, 'You mentioned in a social media post that if you've been dieting half your adult life, you're doing it wrong.' And that was the final nail in her figurative coffin for the diet mentality. I've had multiple people say similar things to me over the years, but she was the first. And without a doubt, she wasn't going to be the last. Luckily, how you approach your nutrition will greatly determine the extent of your results. It starts with rewiring your mindset around the diet mentality.

HOW TO FIX THE DIET MENTALITY

If you want to avoid getting the mumps, you get a shot. If you want to avoid getting rubella, you do the same. Unfortunately, there's no shot that's been designed to avoid getting the diet mentality – not yet anyway – although I secretly hope this book will be the literary equivalent of that. But the inoculation or cure doesn't come in the form of a terrifying needle; it has to do with your mindset. I've broken it down into some easy steps to follow.

1. Cut the word 'diet' from your vocabulary

Or at least change the way you use the word. When I work with clients, we use the term 'nutritional plan' – a nutritional plan includes food items you enjoy, fits into your lifestyle or schedule and is in alignment with your goals. If your goals change, the plan changes, but not drastically. If your goal shifts from reducing body fat to building some lean muscle tissue or 'toning up', then you slightly increase your calorie intake and ensure that you are getting enough amino acids from protein-based foods to adequately repair from your workout sessions. Generally, training would change at such a time too. Instead of cardio or high-intensity interval training (HIIT) at the end of workout, you would want to add a few extra sets of squats.

2. Change your goals

One thing is for certain: when it comes to weight loss, your goals should change! Unless you are severely overweight or morbidly obese, your goal for the next 18 months shouldn't be 'weight loss' or 'fat loss'. If it is, you're doing it wrong. If you're reading this and thinking, 'Oh crap, that's me', don't worry either. We will have it addressed by the end of the book. Again, if that's what you've been doing up until now, that's fine; but now you have feedback that something is wrong with your process. You're not tracking calories, you're not sleeping or recovering well enough, or something similar. But there is a problem that needs to be addressed.

Your goals don't always have to be related to body composition either. Maybe you want to get a bit stronger and hit a personal best on a squat or deadlift or you want to run a 5K, a half marathon or a full marathon. Regardless, apart from the metabolic benefit of not always being in a caloric deficit, the psychological advantage of focusing on a new challenge can support your motivation levels as well.

3. Focus on the process

In Chapter One, I will talk to you about getting your ladder up against the right wall. It basically means that you set the correct goal for yourself and then consider the best approach that will support that end goal. For example, if I want to lose fat, I need to get into a calorie deficit – simple and straightforward. Where this analogy really kicks in is in the 'process' or the figurative climbing of the ladder. A diet is normally outcome-based: I follow this action to get that end result. For example, I will eat salad for every meal because I want to lose 5 kilos. You don't necessarily enjoy the process (eating salad for every meal), but you're willing to sacrifice your happiness or wellbeing for the end goal (losing 5 kilos).

A nutrition-based approach is different. It focuses on both the process *and* the outcome. The outcome or goal doesn't change – you still want to lose 5 kilos – but the way you approach it is different. When it comes to getting rid of the diet mentality, the focus is always on the process, and you regularly need to ask yourself the following two questions:

1. Am I enjoying the process?
2. Is it in alignment with my end goal?

If the answer to both is yes, then you figuratively keep climbing that ladder or to put it literally, you just keep doing what you have been doing. Remember, a diet is restrictive; a nutritional plan isn't. A diet works in the short term; a nutritional plan works for the long term.

How to switch from a 'diet' to a 'nutritional plan'

It's actually relatively simple. As mentioned before, you include food items you enjoy in your plan, and you match it with your goals. Now I'm going to introduce you to a fact that is an underlying theme throughout this book. There is no such thing as 'good' or 'bad' food; food has no morals.

True, there are food items that have higher or lower calorie content, and there are those that have higher or lower nutritional value, but that doesn't make them 'good' or 'bad'. If you're looking to get into a calorie deficit in order to lose fat, a chocolate bar isn't inherently a 'bad' food. It just has more calories and fewer nutrients than, say, a head of broccoli. True, it might not be the most supportive food to include in your plan if you're trying to save on calories, but if it's included in a calorie-controlled plan, where the other 80 per cent of your food is nutrient-dense and you're staying in a calorie deficit, then it's probably fine. Also, if that single food choice, a chocolate bar in this case, is the thing that allows you to stick to your nutritional plan, then I'd make the counter argument that it's a supportive option to include on a daily basis.

Nutritional plan top tips

- **Context matters.** If including your favourite foods helps you stay on the plan, then it's probably a good idea to include them in it.

- **Consistency matters.** If including your favourite foods helps you stick to your plan every day, then it's a probably a good idea to include them consistently every day.

- **Adherence matters.** If including your favourite foods is something you can adhere to over the long term by factoring it into your plan, then it's probably a good idea to include them.

- **Food does not have morals.** Separating foods into 'good' and 'bad' is fine for a five-year-old, but so is believing in Santa Claus and the Tooth Fairy. Just because it was fine when you were a kid, it doesn't make it a good idea for now.

The pyramid of prioritisation

One of my pet peeves when it comes to the 'diet mentality' in the health and fitness industry is the majoring in minor things. A diet example of majoring in minor things is eliminating entire food groups because a 'diet said so'. Two examples of these fashionable weight loss diets are the ketogenic diet, where you greatly reduce all carbs and protein, and the Atkins diet, where you eliminate carbs entirely. To reduce body fat, you need to be in a calorie deficit – no more, no less. The diet you use in order to achieve this is largely irrelevant. It's the mindset you bring to the diet that is going to determine its success.

Personally, I do have a professional preference when it comes to weight-loss nutritional plans: I like to ensure that my clients are in a calorie deficit using nutrient-dense foods such as complete protein sources, healthy fats, complex carbohydrates and plenty of fruits and vegetables, but that's just my philosophy as a coach. You can also lose body fat by getting into a deficit with processed food and chocolate bars, but you just won't feel very good. Your energy levels will be low, and your recovery will be terrible. Additionally, the lack of nutrients will probably reduce your adherence too, so it's not the best option in terms of sustainability. However, once you maintain the deficit, it's still feasible to lose a lot of body fat this way.

But the majoring in minor things brings me to what is probably the most important point when it comes to sustainable fat loss: the pyramid of prioritisation. In other words, what is the one thing you need to do in order to lose fat? What forms the foundation of fat loss and the bottom of the pyramid? That's a calorie deficit. Similar to building a house, the roof and the interior design are all important, but the foundations are what everything else is built upon. Think of your roof as your macro nutrients and the interior design as your food choices. You can have the best roof ever (macros) and a beautiful interior design (food choices) but if there's a rocky foundation (too many calories), it all falls apart.

In the nutritional sense, a focus on macros is useful, but only focusing on protein for bodybuilding or on fat in a keto diet, for example, is a recipe for failure. Food choices are the same. You can eat only 'clean' or healthy foods, but too many calories are too many calories, whatever foods they come from. When it comes to majoring in major things, start with the foundation of your pyramid, calculate your calories and then work your way up. After that, hit your protein requirements to repair. Then, adjust your fat or carbohydrate intake based on your individual preferences or current goals.

- Calories (bottom)
- Macros (middle)
- Food choices (top)

How to stop dieting forever

The pyramid of prioritisation principle is a useful tool to refer to, as it can be adopted regardless of the goal. Whether you're trying to lose fat or build muscle, the same principles apply. Only the specific details will change. As I mentioned earlier, learning how to 'diet' can be a useful skill; just don't confuse it with a lifestyle change. I'll even go as far to say that if you want to keep the word 'diet', do – just ensure that you change your association with it.

The cure for fat loss requires a strong mindset that rewires failure as feedback and allows you to constantly test things out so that you can find what works the best for you.

Again, super simple. But just because it's simple, it doesn't make it easy. Knowing it at least arms you for the battle ahead. After that, it's all about becoming very clear on your end goal or, to use the analogy from earlier, getting your ladder against the right wall.

Getting your ladder against the right wall

Picture this. You are climbing up a ladder placed against a very high wall. It's a scorching hot day and your lips are dry from the heat, but you keep climbing. You put one foot in front of the other, and you continue moving up the ladder. Finally, you're at the top. You look around and think, 'This isn't where I wanted to go … Oh crap, my ladder is up against the wrong wall!'

We have all experienced this kind of feeling in some way or other in our lives. For me, it happened when I was working full time as a primary school teacher in London. I spent four years getting my undergraduate degree, then another full year getting my post-graduate degree. After a year of teaching practice, made up of days of study and sleepless nights, I finally landed a teaching job. I wasn't even an hour into my first day at school when I realised my ladder was against the wrong wall. I had the sinking feeling: This is not what I'm supposed to be doing with my life. I had spent years climbing a ladder, but it was against the wrong wall. This happens to all of us at some stage or another, be it in terms of a career, a romantic relationship or, in the context of this book, the diets you've been following. The problem with climbing a ladder is that it's very difficult to stop yourself from moving up even when you realise you're up against the wrong wall, because the sunk cost fallacy kicks in.

Christopher Olivola, an assistant professor of marketing at Carnegie Mellon's Tepper School of Business, defines the sunk cost effect as 'the general tendency for people to continue an endeavour, or continue consuming or pursuing an option, if they've invested time or money or some resource in it'. He warns, however, that the 'effect becomes a fallacy if it's pushing you to do things that are making you unhappy or worse off'.

This is a common reason why people return to diets that have worked for them in the past. Rather than considering the negative behavioural patterns that get further entangled the more they follow this diet pattern, they justify it with 'Well, it worked last time', or 'I lost 5 kilos when I did it before, so I'll just do it again'. They never think about their future self or consider that once they stop that particular diet, they'll be right back to where they started. It's entirely unrealistic to repeat the same thing over and over again and expect a different result. Now, I won't go as far to say that this is an insane approach, because it's easy to see the logic in this way of thinking, but the next time you find yourself about to behave this way, ask yourself instead: If I follow this diet again, am I just going to end up back where I started six months from now? And now that you've considered that question, let me put another one before you: Why do you think you go back to what you know or to what has worked in the past even though you know deep down that it doesn't work in the long term?

Here's my take on it. It's significantly less demanding to stick with what's familiar, and starting anything new is difficult. It's easier to figuratively climb the ladder that's already against the wrong wall than to pick the ladder up and move it to where it's supposed to be. I get it – I've done it myself.

The very fact that you've picked up this book and are looking for the long-term solution tells me that you have the mindset to get your ladder up against the right wall. Here's the philosophy I use with clients that gets them started on the right foot before embarking on a new nutritional journey. We've already established that starting something new is the hardest part, so this was what I call 'Why going from 0 to 1 is harder than going from 1 to 10', or 'The 0 to 1 principle' for short.

GOING FROM 0 TO 1 VERSUS GOING FROM 1 TO 10

I'm going to start with a story outside of nutrition, but bear with me – it comes full circle. In August 2017, I signed up for the biggest physical challenge of my life: the 2018 Marathon Des Sables – six self-sufficient marathons back-to-back though the Sahara Desert. At that point in my life, I had never run a marathon. Two years before, I was competing as a bodybuilder and finished 8th in the Fitness Model World Championship in Las Vegas. In terms of physical conditioning, I was as far away from a marathon runner as you could be, and when I started training for the Sahara, it showed. I remember my first 2km training run like it was yesterday. I did my normal bodybuilding workout split – chest, shoulders and triceps – and then jumped on a treadmill at the end of my workout. I set the incline to 1.5 and the speed to 15km per hour. At that time, I wasn't aware if 15km per hour was fast or slow, but it was the number I chose. Ten minutes later, my legs felt like jelly and I nearly fell off the treadmill. I thought I was going to get sick. I remember sitting in the changing room after that session, feeling ill to my stomach, thinking, what the f*ck have I just signed up for? Six back-to-back marathons meant 250km, and I was feeling sick after 2km!

At the time, I had to take a long, hard look at the mirror and think about what I had to do in order to achieve this goal. I applied here the same logic behind the nutrition pyramid of prioritisation approach we discussed earlier. I focused on building my fitness to run a single marathon. My thinking was that there's no point worrying about running six marathons if I can't even run a single one. So, I set that as my goal. On the next training day, I did 2km again. It was hard but bearable. For the following three workouts, I did exactly the same. Then, the following week, I increased it to 3km, then the week after to 4km and 5km after that. And that was when something strange happened. I didn't go from 5km to 6km in the natural linear progression. I went from 5km to 10km! Two weeks later, I went from 10km to 20km. My progress wasn't linear. At first it was slow but steady, and then it took what felt like quantum leaps.

Now, as a fitness professional and coach, I am aware that that's not what's going to happen to everybody who sets out on a similar path as me. However, it did make me think about those quantum leaps. And it brought me to the realisation that getting started is the hardest part.

That goes for beginning a new diet or a training programme,

starting a new job or even embarking on a new relationship. You build confidence from competence, and competence comes from experience. When you are going from 0 to 1, you have little experience. So, you have little competence, which leads to little confidence. It sounds so simple, and it is. Yet, when it comes to its application, we tend to forget it.

Let's consider your diet, for example. The temptation is to follow the diet that promises quick and easy results. It's the dietary equivalent of a 'get rich quick' scheme. But as I said earlier, if it sounds too good to be true, it probably is, and that's what every diet that promises you the sun, the moon and the stars is. An advertisement tells you that you can eat as many chocolate cakes and cookies as you want, just take this pill or tea that helps you poop it all out. What they don't advertise is all the other nutrients – you know, the things you need to survive – that get pooped out with it, causing all sorts of adverse side effects. And before you ask, yes, that's a legitimate product that is sold on the market.

What's even more common is an advertisement that asks, 'Do you want to lose weight? Here, just have this bar or drink this shake twice a day and the fat will melt right off.' What they fail to mention is that any massive calorie restriction will have that same impact on weight loss. However, once you go back to eating normal food again, the weight rebounds faster than a jet plane.

It's useful to train yourself to look at the situations above with a sceptical eye. Your default isn't to look for the quick fix. On the contrary, you're suspicious of the quick fix and are always mentally prepared for the hard road. But the hard road is generally the one that leads you to your destination. And as somebody who has walked that road on many occasions, it only looks like the hard road to the people looking in from the outside. Let me explain.

Most people are surprised when I tell them that as a non-runner training for those marathons, running from 2km to 3km was harder than it was running from 10km to 20km. Every one of those 2km runs made me feel sick. And the only reason I didn't go from 10km to more than 20km in one go was because of other time commitments with family and work. This is because the start of any new journey is the most difficult part, then as you get used to it, it becomes your new normal.

Later I speak about the 'ready, aim, fire' approach when it comes to setting any new goal for yourself. The same philosophy can be applied to your diet and nutrition. Pick a plan and just start. You don't need all the calories to be calculated exactly. You don't need the macros down to a tee. You just need to start and course-correct as you go. You can follow the sample plan included in Part Five of this book; alternatively, you can make any weight-loss plan work for you once you consider these basic nutritional principles:

- Have an idea of your calorie intake.
- Use real food more often than not and minimise the intake of processed food.
- Have some form of protein in your major meals.

Then adjust as you go along – if your weight-loss progress is too slow, start tracking your calories more rigidly. If your energy levels are poor, start looking at your actual food choices. Assuming you are sleeping well and eating nutrient-dense foods with lots of green leafy vegetables, energy fluctuations shouldn't be an issue, provided there's no underlying medical condition. If you are not recovering from workouts, look at your protein intake and make sure you are getting enough amino acids (the building blocks of protein) to repair. Starting is the key, but please don't wait a full week, month or year to do so.

THE MYTH OF 'MAGIC MONDAY'

Let me ask you a question. If I arrive at your house on a Wednesday afternoon and tell you there is €100,000 buried under your back lawn, what will you do? Just so we're clear, in this example, it's the truth – no tricks or conspiracy. A satellite signal picked up the treasure chest and it's buried under your lawn. It's on your property, so it's yours to keep. All I am doing is making you aware that it's there. Now, what would you do? Would you wait until Monday to dig it up? F*ck no, you wouldn't wait. You'd grab a shovel and start digging! Now, with that in mind, let me ask you another question.

A nutritionist or dietitian designs a nutritional plan for you on a Wednesday afternoon. When do you honestly think you'll start it? If you're like most people, you'll be excited to start a new plan, motivated to change, and then start on Monday. Why is that? It's another interesting question, and I'm not going to go into the psychological effects of procrastination and immediate gratification, as both are beyond the scope of this book; I'll keep this much more practical. But let's take a step backwards first.

I run my own business, and some people call me a 'lifestyle entrepreneur', which means that all my courses and programmes are based around my own qualifications and interests. I'm a certified personal trainer, strength and conditioning coach and sport nutritionist; therefore, my programmes are designed around those qualifications. My original degree was in business and marketing, so my courses are an amalgamation of that and my experience in running my own online fitness business. The only thing that I'm not technically qualified in, ironically, is writing. Apart from my four years as an English teacher, I have no background in literature and have never taken a course in writing. But here I am, writing books. And between you and me, of all the things I do in my business, it's the most difficult job. Not because I don't love it, I do. I just find it easier to create programmes and courses and to speak. Writing is a struggle for me. That's why I have significantly fewer books than I do courses, programmes and podcast episodes.

Writing books takes a lot more time and effort on my part, but because of this, I have to be very careful not to become complacent. One of my tactics for doing this is to always write when I feel motivated, regardless of where I am in the world. If I'm on a plane and inspiration for a chapter hits me, I start writing on the Notes app on my phone. If I'm mid-workout and more inspiration for the section I was working on the previous day comes to me, I stop and capture it (assuming I'm not training for an event, in which case, I take the hit and miss out on the inspiration). But my reason for doing it is based on the 0 to 1 principle.

Motivation comes and goes; you can't really count on it, but if it comes at the right time, it makes things so much easier. The inspirational or motivating moments pass if you don't take advantage of them at the time, and because I do make the most of those moments, on days I'm not feeling inspired or motivated to write, I have a piece of work to start from rather than trying to go from 0 to 1. Some of the writing I am most proud of has been written midway through a run or in the queue at an airport check-in. But what does that have to do with my diet? The answer is everything. It's exactly the same. Inspiration and motivation are unpredictable in all facets of life, so you need to take advantage of them whenever they show up.

Motivation and your diet

If you're feeling motivated enough to buy a book, sign up with a trainer or pay for a programme, you're feeling pretty damn inspired in that moment. So, why let it fade away to start on Monday? Why not capitalise on the inspiration right now? Why not start, or at least implement, some of the strategies today? What's stopping you? Yes, you might start today and fall off the track tomorrow, but that's why it's so important to be aware of self-sabotage tactics, such as 'pressing the f*ck-it button'. Don't look a gift horse in the mouth. If you feel motivated today, then start today. At least you're moving then. You're getting over that initial difficulty of going from 0 to 1. My first 2km run felt harder than any marathon I've ever run. And that's the truth.

So, I ask you this. The next time you decide you want to lose weight or get in shape, are you going to wait until Monday to start? If you can't give yourself a solid reason, then start today! It's not easy, but it really is that simple.

I'm not very religious, but the 'Last Supper Myth' is what I call the thought process of 'F*ck it, diet starts tomorrow. Let's eat everything in the house tonight.' I understand the epicurean temptation. Tomorrow, I start my weight-loss journey, so tonight we go crazy. I get this more than anyone. Back in 2014, when I used to prepare for fitness model shows, I would routinely have my Last Supper. I would have to mentally prepare myself for 8–12 weeks of eating nothing but chicken, broccoli and rice (which isn't a very sustainable approach obviously), but the night before I planned to start my diet, I would clear the house of all the chocolate, ice-cream and cookies I could lay my hands on. The justification was, 'Well if they're not in the house, they won't tempt me, or I'm not going eat any of these foods for the next few weeks, so I better eat as much as I can before I start my diet tomorrow.' When it's put in writing, it sounds so silly, but it is considerably easier to fall into this trap when it actually happens in your own life. Every time I run one of my online programmes, I inevitably get somebody who mentions or brings up their version of a Last Supper. It's normally accompanied by a photo of a box of cookies, a large tub of ice-cream or a massive Chinese takeaway with captions such as 'Getting rid of all this before the six weeks start' or some variation of that. My reply is nearly always the same: why? Where is the food going tomorrow? Has the world stopped making cookies?

This normally opens up a dialogue in which the person claims they can't have the food in their house because it will end up tempting them, and I get that. Sometimes having a good preventive system in place is a good strategy over using your own willpower, but it is not so always. Yet, it's still a meaningful question. Where is the food going tomorrow? It's still going to be available in shops. You're probably still going to walk past it on your next grocery shop outing. The chocolate, cake or biscuit industry didn't decide they're just going to shut down because you've decided you want to lose weight. So, what's the solution? Simple. Don't reject your favourite foods. Understand that they're probably more calorific and less nutrient-dense than some alternatives, but that's it. Also, eating everything in sight before you start on a weight-loss journey is like learning to drive with a blindfold on. Technically, you might drive from destination A to destination Z unharmed, but my money is on you crashing before making it to destination B or C. The Last Supper mindset has you eating everything in sight because you think those food items will be off limits until you hit your weight-loss goal, but you'll see why that just isn't the case.

On top of that strategy being unhelpful when it comes to food relationships, it also doesn't make any practical sense when it comes to basic caloric intake. Let's take your money for example. Your goal is to save more money. Now say you saved €10 six days of the week for a total of €60 but on day seven, you spent €100. What happened? You're down €40 at the end of the week. Your bank balance doesn't care how 'good' you were the other six days; all it cares about is what's in your account at the end of the week. In this case, it's negative €40. Your calories are the same. If you're undereating during the week and then bingeing during the weekend, that's putting you into a calorie surplus and your waistline won't care how many salads you had for lunch Monday to Friday. All it sees is a calorie surplus, and calorie surplus = weight gain.

Now apply the Last Supper theory to this. If you massively overeat the day or the weekend before you start a new nutritional plan, do you think your waistline cares that you're starting a 'diet' from the next day? No, it doesn't. There are two main ways to address the Last Supper problem. The first is mentioned above. You have to understand basic caloric balance. Think of the minus

€40 in your bank account. The second is to stop separating food into categories of good and bad – remember, food has no morals. For now, if you're tempted to have the Last Supper before you get started on the plan from this book, nip that unsupportive idea in the bud right now. If you want to have ice-cream every day and you factor it into your calorie intake, then that's what you do.

FINDING YOUR 'WHY'

I want to introduce you to two of my previous clients, Jack and Kate. Jack is 32 years old, works in an office nine to five, Monday to Friday, and wants to lose about 5 kilos. Kate is the same age and works in the office across the street. She too wants to lose about 5 kilos. Jack comes to me and says, 'Brian, I need to lose 5 kilos.' My follow-up question, which has been the same for over 10 years, is, 'Okay, why do want to lose 5 kilos?' Then the conversation goes like this:

Jack: Because I need to lose 5 kilos.
Me: Okay, I get that Jack, but why do you want to lose 5 kilos?
Jack: I have it to lose.
Me: Hmmmmm.
Now Kate arrives. Same problem, same question.
Me: Okay Kate, why do you want to lose 5 kilos?
Kate: Well, I have my sister's wedding coming up in two months.
Me: Okay, why do you want to lose 5 kilos for your sister's wedding in two months, Kate?
Kate: There's a dress that I really want to fit into.
Me: Why do you want to fit into the dress?

Kate: I don't know, I'll just feel more confident and eh ... sexier if I can fit into it …

Me: Cool, why do you want to feel more confident and sexier at the wedding?

Kate: Well, actually, a guy I really fancy is going to be there.

Me: Got it.

Now, with an objective lens, who do you think is going to have a better chance at hitting their 5 kilo weight-loss target? Jack, who wants to lose 5 kilos because 'he has it to lose' or Kate who wants to lose 5 kilos so she can feel more confident and sexier in front of someone she's attracted to? You got it. Kate is going to win this race every day of the week. But why? Over the years, I've had countless variations of this same conversation, but the end message never changes. You need to know why you're doing what you're doing. You need to find your why! Why do you want to lose weight? Why do you want to look a certain way? For this, I normally apply the 'ask why – rule of three' technique. Ask why three times until you get to the root of why you're doing something. You may find the answer after asking it once or you may need to ask why more than three times, but most people tend to get to the root of why they want to lose weight after they ask themselves three times. In case you were wondering, Kate did lose her 5 kilos for the wedding. To be fair, Jack did too, but it took him much longer, and until we found the root of why he wanted to lose weight, the scale kept rebounding up and down. That's normally what happens, and the same thing will happen to you if you don't question why you're doing it in the first place. 'I want to lose 5 kilos' is a better goal than 'I want to lose weight' –

at least its more specific. But it's still not deep enough to sustain you on your journey of weight loss.

So ask yourself: do you want to lose weight so that you feel sexier? Do you want to lose weight because you fear for your health? Do you want to lose weight so that you can move around and play with your kids, nieces or nephews? Finding your why will help you more than any number that is reflected back at you on a weighing scale.

Believe it or not, 99 per cent of the people I've worked with – who listed weight loss as their primary goal – thought that losing weight was what they wanted to achieve. It wasn't. In reality, that was just an external representation of the emotion they were looking to induce because of their association with a certain level of body composition. Or because they felt lonely, unconfident or unattractive, and they thought that losing weight would stop them from feeling that way. Unfortunately, that's not always the case. Unless you are somebody who is clinically overweight or obese, whose quality of life will dramatically improve from losing weight, the larger majority is stuck in the 'I'll be happy when' fallacy: 'I'll be happy when I lose X amount of weight', 'I'll be happy when I get to Y dress size' or 'I'll be happy when I look a certain way'. The truth is, most people desire a feeling, not a number on a scale, and being aware of that is the first step on the ladder against the right wall. Before long-term weight loss can be achieved, you need to figure out what the feeling is that you're looking to minimise or eliminate.

This book will be your A-to-Z guide on how to lose weight and reduce body fat. You track your calories and get into a caloric deficit; you do that with foods you enjoy – it really is that simple.

Then, why is it so difficult to actually do it? Sometimes it's down to all the misinformation that's out there, which I will hopefully address, but there's also the emotional side to consider when long-term weight loss is the goal. Losing 5 kilos doesn't mean you'll feel more confident. It certainly increases the chances for it to happen and how you lost the weight can either build or destroy confidence, but it's no guarantee. The only guarantee when you lose 5 kilos is that you will weigh 5 kilos less when you step on a scale. Everything else – how you feel, the confidence you build and so on – will all be determined by how you hit your end goal, not by the achievement of the end goal itself. Consider these two scenarios:

1. Alison goes on an extreme calorie-restricted plan. It's a bar-and-juice-only diet, where she eats or drinks 600–1,000kcal every day. Alison has some lapses, where she binges and eats everything in sight, but for the most part, she sticks to it. Over the course of six weeks, she loses 5 kilos.

2. Seán goes into a slight calorie deficit, exercises a little more, and loses 5 kilos over a similar timeframe.

Are both those scenarios the same? No, but the end results look the same. That's where the confusion arises from. From the outside, both Alison and Seán have lost 5 kilos. They have the same objective end result, but their processes were completely different. Let's look at these examples from a different perspective.

Who do you think is going to have more confidence after losing the 5 kilos? Is it Alison, who jumped on a quick-fix solution without altering any non-supportive behaviours or educating themselves on the basic principles of nutrition? Or is it Seán, the person who had to make small lifestyle adjustments and incorporated new supportive habits to hit the same end goal? The answer is pretty obvious: Seán is going to feel much better about himself. But why is that?

WHY THE PROCESS MATTERS

There are two ways to set goals. One is outcome driven, and the other is process driven. Outcome-driven goals are just as they sound. They are all about the outcome. For example, 'I want to lose 5 kilos, and I don't care what I have to do to get there. As long as I lose 5 kilos, I'll be content.'

Process-driven goals are different. They take the end goal into consideration as well – they always keep the end in mind – but they give equal, if not more thought to the actual process. How they hit their end goal matters a great deal. One of my mentors used to say – albeit in relation to business advice – that losers focus on outcome-driven goals and winners focus on process-driven goals. To help us better understand this, let's go back to our ladder analogy.

In an outcome-driven goal, you would see the rooftop (or losing 5 kilos) as the end goal. You put on the blinkers and climb the ladder, never focusing or questioning any of the individual steps of the ladder. You just keep going. The diet equivalent is just following some fad or trend because it's easy to do and you don't really have to understand it. Popular or trendy diets, as their name suggests, are relatively straightforward to follow. You don't need to educate yourself on basic nutrition; just do 'X', and you get 'Y' – just drink this 600kcal-a-day shake and lose 5 kilos. But in reality, you should question anything that sounds like a quick fix. These types of diets are always marketed as outcome driven. If they talked about the process, how you'd be hungry, moody, lethargic or, worse, nutrient deficient with potential long-term consequences, the diet wouldn't sound half as appealing. It sounds like common sense, but unfortunately common sense isn't so common now, with the power of marketing, branding or the emotional manipulating that leads us into easing a pain point with a quick-fix solution. I've fallen for them myself, and the temptation never goes away – you just become better at filtering through the nonsense.

So, that's the outcome-driven goal. Now, let's look at how somebody with a process-driven mindset would approach it. Someone with a process-driven goal would do it differently. On each rung of the ladder, they would ask themselves, 'Am I enjoying this process?' They would have the end goal in mind (the rooftop or losing 5 kilos), but they would also pause and reflect on how they were getting there. If they were starving, moody and lethargic all the time, that would be feedback that the process they had chosen clearly wasn't sustainable for them. Again, failure isn't final; it's feedback. But you have to incorporate that feedback into what you do next in order to succeed. A quote regularly attributed to Buddha goes, 'If you can't be happy on the journey, how do you expect to be happy when you reach the destination?', and weight loss is a lot like that. Sure, you can drink 600kcal of a juice every day for six weeks, but could you do it for six months, six years? Probably not. This fails the process test immediately. But could you calculate your calories and eat slightly under your maintenance with foods you enjoy for six weeks? What about six months or six years? You probably could. As I mentioned earlier, if your goal has been weight loss for the last six years, you're doing something wrong, as your goals should change regularly; but I think the six-year example helps illustrate my point here.

Although this book is about nutrition, it relates somewhat to personal development as well: if you're trying to lose weight, you're trying to develop yourself personally; your physical appearance is just the current manifestation of that. And that's why it's so important to consider your mindset too. The simple equation I regularly gave my clients is weight loss - mindset = upset.

HOW TO AVOID THE MINDSET PITFALLS IN WEIGHT LOSS

1. Focus on the process and make sure your ladder is up against the right wall.

2. Ask why three times: why do you want to lose weight, reduce body fat or look a certain way? Write your answers down in a journal.

3. Keep your comparisons realistic. Compare against yourself but be realistic about what it took to get you there.

4. DON'T compare yourself with others.

The last point above about comparison is an entire book in itself, but how you compare is important. You should compare yourself with yourself. Are you improving? Are you losing weight? Is your sleep getting better this month? Did you make better food choices this week compared to last week? Are you getting better? These are all very useful questions to ask. However, comparing yourself with that social media model or the physically attractive person in your local gym is a recipe for misery. Not only is it generally not helpful, unless you're taking inspiration from them, it's also not very practical. This is your story, not theirs.

Now, this begs the next logical question: how do I start and where do I go from here? Well, let's get into that now. I've mentioned 'ready, aim, fire' when it comes to setting any new goal for yourself. Now, I'm going to flip that slightly and tell you about an even more effective method for weight loss. I call it 'ready, fire, aim'.

Ready, fire, aim, and the curse of the 'perfect' time

I need to get a new pair of running shoes before I start running. I need to do an overhaul on my diet if I want to lose weight. It's New Year's Day – I need to sign up to a gym straight away! AND I'll buy a membership for the entire year. If I pay for it, I'll definitely use it, right? Does any of this sound familiar? I'm not going to tell you I haven't done this; I can veer towards 'paralysis by analysis' tendencies myself, i.e., overthinking an entire situation until I've sufficiently freaked myself out to the point that I don't take any action. If that's you or you're a procrastinator who is always waiting for the right day, time or place to start something new, then the 'ready, fire, aim' technique might be a useful approach for you. It's exactly as it sounds, too. You get ready (set the goal), fire (start moving towards the goal) and aim (course-correct if you're going wrong).

It sounds so obvious when I put it like that, but that's not generally how we approach the goals we set for ourselves. Most of us hate uncertainty, and having all our ducks in a row allows us to feel like we're making the best use of our time when, in fact, we would have been better off just starting with less information and course-adjusting as went along. If you want to lose weight, it's easy to focus on all the changes you need to make: a completely new diet plan, a brand-new workout regimen, and maybe even a personal trainer in your local gym to keep you accountable. That's all well and good, but it's generally not the most effective way to lose weight over the long term. The most efficient way is to incorporate a minimum effective dose (MED) approach in everything fitness-related in your life.

If you're not currently working out or have never followed an exercise regimen, start by adding a couple of workouts a week. Don't change your food, don't hire a coach. Just make this one small change, but make sure you stick to it. For 99 per cent of people, changing this one variable and keeping everything else the same will elicit weight loss (as you'll be burning more calories each day). Then, if and when that plateaus, look at your nutrition.

Again, no overhaul – just small, simple changes. You normally have cereal, toast and jam for breakfast. Cool, switch to porridge for the next week. Keep your lunch and dinner the same. Then, after a week, look at making healthier choices for your lunch. Instead of white bread, ham and a chocolate bar, try wholegrain or sourdough bread, chicken and an apple. Keep dinner the same as always. Then, after another week, look at your dinner. Instead of a burger and chips, make some oven-baked homemade French fries and use lean mince for your burger. No crazy dramatic changes, just small ones each week. If these changes are the only ones you make, you'll see a drastic difference in your waistline by the end of the month. Not only that, but the changes are so small that you probably won't even notice that, in the space of a month, you go from not exercising and making poor food choices to working out a few times a week and eating a good-quality breakfast, lunch and dinner.

Making too many changes all at once is a recipe for failure from the get-go. Instead of making all these drastic changes up front, which sets most people up to fail, start small (ready), try simple changes (fire) and then make bigger changes as you go along (aim).

Obviously, if you want more drastic results, you make bigger changes, but the principle is the same. You don't start training for your first marathon by running 26.2 miles all at once. You start by running 1 mile, then 2 miles, then 3 miles and so on, until you get to where you can run 26.2 miles. Your nutrition is exactly the same. It's vital to always keep the end goal in mind, but it's equally important to focus on how you can WIN, or the 'what's important now?' principle. What can you do today or right now that will help you with the end goal?

Apply the WIN principle and ask yourself, 'What's important now?' then do just that. Personally, as an endurance athlete, speaker and author, I know that I can't make massive changes and stick to them long term. Even while writing this book (and my past books), I followed this 'ready, fire, aim' approach – otherwise, I would never start writing. So, I just sit and write, and I course-correct as I go along. Sometimes my writing is garbage, and I'd be embarrassed if anybody saw it. Other times, it feels inspired – like somebody else took over my body – and I think, I can't believe I wrote that. It just came flowing out. But 100 per cent of the time, I just turn up and write. If it's good, great. If it's not, I can always change it.

Your fitness journey is exactly the same. Don't wait for Monday to start a new workout regimen; start today (or tomorrow at the latest) and get moving. If you need to adjust the workouts as you go, that's fine, but get started. Don't wait for New Year's or till after the Saturday night party to go on a diet. If you want to lose weight, get into a calorie deficit now and then course-correct for Saturday. If it's Thursday, eat fewer calories that day and the next day, enjoy the party on Saturday, and then go back to a calorie deficit on Sunday. No fuss, no muss – best of all worlds.

I also used the 'ready, fire, aim' philosophy when I started training to run 230km through the Arctic Circle in February 2019. I dedicated hours to training, got to know what foods wouldn't freeze at −38 °C, and headed to the Arctic. At 86km from the finish line, I tore my Achilles tendon (the one on the back of your foot, just above your heel and below your calf). One thing these challenges have taught me about life is that the world doesn't give a f*ck about your plan. You want to run 230km in the Arctic, cool, you can train and plan all you want, but here's a torn Achilles tendon 86km from the end, deal with that, bro! You can plan for the best, but you need to be mentally prepared for the worst. That's why your mindset is so important. So if you fall off your diet, you deal with it then. As you'll see later, it's not about how you feel in the moment; it's about asking yourself what your target self would do. For now, your target self is just the person you want to become in the future.

- My target self knows that pain is temporary, and it will eventually go away.
- My target self knows that the hardest part of any new goal is the beginning.

- My target self knows that if I overthink things, I won't even get started.

But what does your target self *do*? Setting goals isn't normally the difficult part. Anybody can say they want to lose weight, they want to run a 10K or they want to squat X amount of weight. It's easy to say it. Actually going and doing it is an entirely different beast – that's why training yourself to do difficult things makes life easier. Remember: ready, fire, aim! The good news is that if you adopt this strategy, it's inevitable that things will feel much easier as the compound effect kicks in.

The compound effect

Darren Hardy, author of *The Compound Effect*, defines it as 'the strategy of reaping huge rewards from small, seemingly insignificant actions'. Just to give you an idea of the power of compounding, here's one of my favourite examples from Hardy's book, called 'the magic penny'. The scenario goes like this: if you were given a choice to receive one million euro in one month or a cent that doubled every day for 30 days, which would you choose? When I first read that, it sounded like a trick question – so I knew that the cent that doubled every day must be the better choice. However, I didn't immediately realise how much better it would be! The following is the calculation for the cent doubling every day:

Day 1: €0.01

Day 2: €0.02

Day 3: €0.04

Day 4: €0.08

Day 5: €0.16

Day 6: €0.32

Day 7: €0.64

Day 8: €1.28

Day 9: €2.56

Day 10: €5.12

Day 11: €10.24

Day 12: €20.48

Day 13: €40.96

Day 14: €81.92

Day 15: €163.84

Day 16: €327.68

Day 17: €655.36

Day 18: €1,310.72

Day 19: €2,621.44

Day 20: €5,242.88

Day 21: €10,485.76

Day 22: €20,971.52

Day 23: €41,943.04

Day 24: €83,886.08

Day 25: €167,772.16

Day 26: €335,544.32

Day 27: €671,088.64

Day 28: €1,342,177.28

Day 29: €2,684,354.56

Day 30: €5,368,709.12

The difference is quite significant. Nothing dramatic really starts to happen until day 18; then the principal grows exponentially. The above example shows you the power of compounding in the investment world, but let's see how compounding works in an everyday scenario.

I want to introduce to three friends: Linda, Sarah and Mary. They're all married and live in the same small town. They also have very similar backgrounds, intelligence levels and personalities. Each makes about €50,000 a year. They have an average health and body weight composition, plus a little bit of that dreaded belly fat. Linda, friend number one, plods along in life, doing what she's always done. She's happy, or thinks she is, but regularly complains that nothing ever really changes or improves in her life.

Sarah, friend number two, starts making some small and seemingly inconsequential positive changes in her life. She begins reading a chapter from a nutritional book or listening to an audiobook for 30 minutes on her commute to work. She wants to improve her life but doesn't want to make a fuss about it or do anything too drastic. She chooses to make some simple changes that can improve her life. A nutrition book she recently read informed her that cutting 125kcal from her diet every day might help her lose a bit of fat around her tummy. I'm talking 125kcal a day, not gradually decreasing it every day. Just a once-off decision, no big deal. That means cutting down a cup of cereal in the morning or trading a can of soda for water at lunchtime. She's also decided to take the stairs at work from now on and skip using the lift. Again, a very simple change – something anyone can do. She is determined to stick with these choices, knowing that even though they're simple, she can easily be tempted to abandon them. Sarah has made the commitment that the changes are non-negotiable – she's doing them whether she feels like it or not.

Mary, friend number three, makes a few poor choices. She recently bought memberships to several online streaming sites to watch more of her favourite shows. She's also been trying out the recipes from the new dessert book she bought. Furthermore, she's decided to frequent the new coffee shop beside her workplace and add a chocolate macchiato to her lunch every day. Black coffee is boring, and she wants to spice it up a little. Nothing crazy, just a small change here and there.

At the end of six months, no perceivable difference exists among the three women. Sarah continues to read a little bit every night and listen to audiobooks during her commute. Mary is 'enjoying' life and doing less. Linda keeps doing what she's always done. Although each has their own pattern of behaviour, six months isn't long enough to see any real decline or improvement in their situations. True, Sarah may look a little leaner and Mary a little heavier, but the changes are hardly noticeable.

Fast forward 18 months and Sarah looks leaner and is clearly more confident. She's read nearly 10 nutrition, health and fitness books over the past 18 months and has been utilising the tips to improve the quality of her life.

Mary is very obviously putting on extra weight. Although she's caught up on her favourite TV shows, she hasn't progressed at work the slightest bit.

Linda is in the same place as she was before.

At the end of 25 months, we start seeing measurable, visible differences in the women. At month 27, the difference is expansive. By month 31, the change is startling! Mary is now overweight, while Sarah is slim. By simply cutting 125 calories a day, in 31 months, Sarah has lost 15 kilos.

31 months = 940 days
940 days @ 125kcal/day = 117, 500 calories
117,500 calories/7,700kcal per kilo = 15.23 kilos

Mary, who consumed 125 more calories a day during the same time, gained 15 kilos! She now weighs 30 kilos *more* than Sarah!

What about Linda? Well, Linda is pretty much exactly where she was two-and-a-half years ago, except more bitter about her situation, as other people have improved their lives while she's still in the same place and looks exactly the same as she did 25 months ago (albeit a little older).

This is a fictitious story, of course, but it illustrates how making small and seemingly insignificant changes can lead to lasting results over time. At this point, you might be thinking, 'I can't wait 25 months! Are you crazy? I need to lose weight now.' So, what do you do if you want results faster? Easy – make more drastic changes. As long as what you're doing is sustainable and aligned with your specific goal, the rate or amount of the change you make is very much down to your personal preference and personality type. Just make sure it is sustainable and you can stick to it. There's a reason you learn to walk before you can run. If you try and run before you know how to walk, you are more likely to fall. When weight loss is the goal, sustainability is the key.

Tell me what you do every day, and I'll tell you where you'll be in a year. Note: I didn't say tell me how you feel every day or tell me what you do on the days you feel motivated. There's a big difference, as I'll explain.

Motivation vs habits

'I'm not feeling very motivated today.'

'That person is so motivated. It's easier for them.'

'If I could just get motivated, then I'd be able to get fitter, lose weight, get stronger.'

If you have ever uttered those words, this next section is for you. Motivation is a great thing to get, but it's not something you always have. There's no such thing as a 'motivated' person! There are disciplined people. There are people who have good daily habits. There are dedicated people.

Motivation is something that comes and goes; although it's great when it does arrive, it determines about 1 per cent of your overall success. The other 99 per cent is down to just showing up and doing what you have to do. My daughter Holly is six years old; so, for the past few Christmases, we've spent the month of December preparing for Santa Claus: picking out the perfect carrot for Rudolph and debating what cookies to leave out for him. I tried to convince her to leave out a chocolate bar this past year instead, but I was overruled. 'Don't be silly. Santa eats *cookies*, Daddy!'. How do you argue about that with a six-year-old? She did have a good point, but I just don't like cookies. Anyway, the beauty of Santa Claus (or birthdays, if you don't celebrate Christmas) is that you know exactly in advance when the arrival is. On the 24th of December, every Christmas Eve, Santa Claus pops down your chimney to distribute toys. You can set your watch to it; you can plan for it, and you know it's coming.

Motivation, on the other hand, is the complete opposite. It can come at any time. Motivation is like the wind for a paddle boat. Your paddling of the boat is your dedication, your discipline and your habits. If a gust of wind comes, that's motivation. It's great when it comes and you can just sit back and enjoy the ride, but there's no guarantee that it's going to come, since you can't control it. But what you *can* control is your paddling, i.e., what you do every day – hitting your daily step count, getting your workout in, making better food choices and so on. So, the question shouldn't be 'How do I get motivated?'; it should be 'How can I build habits that make my life better?'. I mention on my podcast regularly that people don't decide their future – they decide their habits, and their habits decide their future. When I started training to run six back-to-back marathons in the Sahara in 2018, I couldn't rely on motivation to do my training sessions. I hated (and still hate) long-distance running, so there were very few things that would help me get motivated to complete a 20km training run. I could preload a YouTube motivational clip or save a favourite podcast to listen to, but that would just make the workout bearable, without me ever really enjoying it. However, the end goal was to run through the Sahara, and to do that, I needed to run every day.

I've already mentioned setting goals using the ready, fire, aim approach. Since I knew this was my goal, now it was a case of building habits that supported it. For me, I still wanted to weight train as normal, so I started getting up at 5 a.m. instead of 6 a.m. I still wanted quality time with my loved ones, so I would shower straight after my training sessions and get directly to work so I could finish my work for the day earlier. Like everybody, there were days when I felt more motivated than others. If I had a rest on the day prior or ate my bodyweight in chocolate, then I would be normally ready to run the following day; but I couldn't rely on that.

Motivation, like the wind, could show up, but what happens when it doesn't? Do you just quit training? Do you just decide not to make a healthier food choice? Do you just go to bed any time you want because you're not feeling 'motivated'? Is that what your target self would do? F*ck no, it isn't; so, you shouldn't either! The next time you feel 'unmotivated', by all means, use the tools mentioned above to get you going. However, don't confuse that with actual progress. Don't confuse paddling with the gusts of wind. The next time you feel 'unmotivated', ask yourself, how can I WIN (what's important now)? Then, do that. If it means listening to your favourite song to get you moving, then that's what you do. If it means re-listening to a health or fitness podcast to get your head straight, then that's what you do. You get the idea.

Use motivational strategies as tools in your arsenal but realise that the concept of 'motivation' or 'motivated people' is absolute horsesh*t when you think about it. Everybody feels motivated some days and unmotivated on others. That's human nature. But don't let how you feel determine what you do. One of my mentors always told me that 'Successful people do what they have to do, whether they feel like it or not.' Santa Claus is reliable. Your birthday is reliable. Motivation isn't, so stop relying on it. Focus on your daily habits instead.

Tell me what you do every day, and I'll tell you where you'll be in a year

Some psychologists believe that up to 90 per cent of our behaviours are habitual. From the time you get up in the morning to the time you retire at night, you do hundreds of things the same way every day – the way you shower, dress, eat, check your phone, brush your teeth, drive or commute to work, organise your desk, shop at the supermarket or clean your bedroom or your house.

The reason the title of this section is effective – and I've mentioned it in the discipline ingredient on page 4 – is because it is applicable to everything we do. Tell or show me how you eat every day and the food choices you make, and I'll tell you how much weight you will lose in a year. Tell me how many steps you do every day or the intensity of your workouts in the gym or at home, and I'll tell you how fit you'll be in a year. It works equally in reverse. For example, if you are consistently eating low-nutrient and high-calorie food, there's a pretty good chance that you're going to be carrying around a spare tyre this time next year. Remember the example of Mary and the compound effect earlier? The beauty of habits is that once you recognise you've created an unsupportive or 'bad' habit, you can change it. It's not necessarily easy to alter, and the deeper engrained it is or the longer you've been doing it, the more difficult it is to change, but it can definitely be done.

I categorise habits into supportive (good) and unsupportive (bad). Supportive habits are the ones that get you closer to your weight-loss goal every single day. If a current habit isn't moving you closer to your weight-loss target, then you need to look at ways to break or change it. I'll start with an extreme example but I think it helps to illustrate my point on how to go about changing or altering unsupportive habits. If somebody is looking to lose 10 kilos but they get a Chinese takeaway four nights a week, it's probably not going to help their weight-loss goal. Straightforward enough. Therefore, they need to change their actions around this unsupportive habit. The first thing is to go from eating

Chinese four nights a week to three nights a week. Assuming they're replacing it with a more supportive food choice, they'll instantly be consuming less calories. They also didn't go from eating Chinese four nights a week to zero nights a week, as that's generally too much of a shock to the system for most people to stick to. Although the temptation is to go cold turkey in contrast to gradually cutting back or focusing on moderation, that's not always the best way to approach it.

Now that they've gone from four nights a week to three nights a week, can you guess what I'm going to recommend next? You got it! Now they reduce it to two nights a week and then once a week and, if they really want to drop the bad habit, eventually to zero nights a week. Again, at this point, if they're factoring it into their overall calorie requirements for the week, they're probably going to be fine having it once a week (especially if they love it); however, four times a week just isn't supportive for a weight loss goal. Quantity matters; so, keep that in mind.

If that example is completely foreign to you, you're probably thinking, 'But I don't eat Chinese four times a week, I think I'm doing everything right but I still can't lose fat from my stomach' – then look at the section on the Seven Deadly Diet Sins and see if you are falling for one or more of those sins.

However, if the above example connects with you, albeit with another food or drink choice – chocolate, ice-cream, beer, wine, crisps, etc., now you might be thinking 'But I want results faster. If I go cold turkey and just drop the Chinese, surely that's going to be better?' Well, that depends. When you are trying to break any bad dietary habit, you really have two options. First, go cold turkey, just give up the food in question, and see if you can stick to it. Second, gradually reduce your intake week by week – as I outlined above – and see how your body fat levels respond.

Self-awareness is the key in choosing the strategy, as some people do better with option one while others do better with option two. I've always been an 'all-or-nothing' person and don't do great with moderation. I generally fare better with abstaining for a given period of time when trying to break a bad habit. Find out what method works best for you.

I am often asked how I know if I should go cold turkey or practise moderation; instead of explaining it in detail, I want to introduce you to a young married couple, Aoife and Carl. Aoife and Carl are on a journey to lose weight. They have decent nutrition and training habits; both go to the gym a few times a week and make good food choices for the most part. But they have the same problem – both of them love chocolate! They are aware that their love of chocolate is probably their main hindrance in losing the desired amount of body fat. So, I want to create a new habit that supports their end goal. Aoife, as we know, has a sweet tooth, and the thought of not having a small bit of chocolate every day makes her physically anxious. Having a chocolate bar at lunchtime is the food highlight of her day, and she looks forward to it all morning. The thought of giving it up or waiting a full week for it makes life unbearable for her (again, I'm being dramatic, but stick with me here).

In this case, Aoife is probably going to be better off eating a little bit of chocolate every day and factoring it into her nutritional strategy. If she manages her calorie and food intake, she can adjust it to fit in a daily bar. As long as she's not consuming too many calories (calorie surplus) and is instead making supportive food choices the rest of the day, despite a chocolate bar every afternoon, her body fat will gradually come down. Such a strategy is going to allow her to adhere to her nutritional plan over the long term, creating a habit that allows her to continually reduce her body fat until she's happy with how she looks.

On the other hand, Carl is a bit more extreme by nature. He wants to get his body fat down as well, but he looks at Aoife and thinks, 'How does she do that? I couldn't eat a small amount of chocolate every day. If I did, I would want to eat the whole box! Besides, I'd rather not have any all week and then have as much as I want during the weekend.' Aoife feels the opposite. She looks at Carl and thinks, 'I couldn't go a whole week without chocolate. I don't know how he does it!' Sound familiar? If you have ever tried to lose weight or reduce body fat, you'll be familiar with such a scenario in some form. Again, it may be with another food or drink of your choice, but the idea is generally the same. At this juncture, you will also connect more with either Aoife or Carl and think one way is better than the other. In the context of getting body fat down, both strategies work. Yes, the tactics may differ, but both work. Aoife has to keep her calories in check each day to factor in her chocolate bar. Carl, conversely, is more likely to reduce his calorie intake in his other meals during the weekends in order to enjoy the several bars he plans to eat on Saturday nights. Regardless, both strategies work. Understanding what tactics you should employ is down to your personality type. Finding what you can stick to is ultimately the end goal.

Take Action

Sit down and really think about where you can make some small changes:

- If your downfall is snacking, do you need to prepare your meals in advance?

- If you keep missing workouts, do you need to get up a little earlier to work out tomorrow?

- If you're often tired, do you need to skip that movie on TV so you can prioritise your sleep tonight?

Self-sabotage

Have you ever uttered the words, 'I know what I need to do, but I just can't do it?'; 'I know I should make healthier food choices, but those biscuits look really tasty right now,' or 'I know I should go for that walk after work but it's cold, wet and windy outside.' If education or knowing was enough, self-sabotage wouldn't be an issue for any of us. It's interesting because at this point in the book, you're probably very clear on what it is you have to do in order to lose weight: get into a calorie deficit, include in your meal plan food items that you enjoy, and make sure the regime is something you can stick to. But we all know it's just not that easy. Up to this point, we have talked about why your mindset is the real secret to making long-term weight loss possible. Now we're going to talk about the 250-kilo gorilla in the room: the self-sabotage mindset. The first step in dealing with self-sabotage is learning to rewire failure as feedback, which we've already discussed at the beginning of the book. Now comes the cherry on top: learning to rest and taking a break or resetting instead of quitting!

Quitting because you are on the wrong path is completely different from quitting because something has become too difficult. The primary reason I speak about 'getting your ladder up against the right wall' earlier in the book is because once you understand the importance of that, the answer to what you should do next becomes much clearer. If your ladder is not up against the right wall and you are following an unsustainable diet and training programme, you won't get results. But once you have a nutritional plan that is sustainable for you, the mindset tools we are going to go through now can eliminate self-sabotage, making it a thing of the past. It starts with why I dislike diets.

WHY I DISLIKE DIETS SO MUCH

Diets are a funny thing, and as you already know, I've never been a fan of the word. For me, a 'diet' is something you follow until you hit a specific goal and then you go back to eating normally. The word by its very nature embodies short-term thinking, which makes it apt for self-sabotage. I've always preferred the term 'nutritional plan', which just refers to the way you eat. However, it's not random – it's specific. Remember, random eating + random training = random results.

If your goal is to lose weight, then a nutritional plan is specific to that. If your goal is to build muscle or get leaner, then your nutritional plan is specific to that. If your goals change, you adjust your nutritional plan – you don't need to do a full overhaul. For example, if your goal shifts from weight loss to toning up or building muscle, you slightly increase your calorie intake and bump up your protein consumption. Conversely, if your goal shifts from toning up and building muscle to losing weight or reducing body fat, you reduce your calorie intake slightly. No overhaul, nothing drastic – just minor alterations. For it to be the perfect nutritional plan that won't lead to self-sabotage, it needs to follow these three criteria:

1. Includes foods you enjoy.
2. Aligns with your goals.
3. Can be adhered or stuck to.

After that, it's really up to you what you do. In my 10 years of working in the fitness and diet industry, it's the only tried-and-tested nutritional approach I've seen. You can make any diet fit it once you've adopted that mindset. From this point on, it's about conditioning yourself to check in on why you keep falling off your plan and how to get back on track if you do go off the rails. I like to call this my one-two punch of:

1. Don't press the f*ck-it button! BUT …
2. Reset it if you do.

1. Don't press the f*ck-it button!

'It's the weekend. F*ck it, I'll eat what I want.'

'It's my sister's wedding. F*ck it, she only gets married once (hopefully), I'll eat what I want.'

'There's ice-cream in the fridge. F*ck it, it's Friday, and I'm tired. I'll just eat what I want.'

'The moons of Jupiter are orbiting a weird way today. F*ck it, I'll eat what I want.'

Does this sound familiar? Is your f*ck-it button completely worn out? Now this isn't to be confused with 'Don't eat certain foods'. As you already know, I'm a big proponent of eating pizza, drinking beer or having that bar of chocolate if that's what allows you to stick to your nutritional plan in the long term. But don't eat the whole pizza. Don't drink 10 beers. Don't eat the family-sized box of chocolates. If losing weight or improving your body composition is your goal, the danger is really in the dosage and the quantity.

An average-sized chocolate bar isn't necessarily a 'bad' food in relation to calories; it has about 230kcal per bar. If you have an allowance of 1,600kcal a day, that's only a small portion of it. However, 10 chocolate bars is 2,300kcal. That puts you into a massive calorie surplus, which will probably lead to weight gain.

However, if you find that you've fallen off the wagon, then it could be time to rest and reset, not quit. Just because you made a few poor choices on a Friday night doesn't mean that it has to roll over the entire weekend. And, if you've had a poor weekend, that doesn't need to throw you off for the entire week or even the following month. If you feel like you have to quit, either you haven't learnt to rest and reset, or your ladder is up against the wrong wall and the unsustainability factor is the reason you can't stick to your plan. Both give you feedback.

- If you haven't learnt to rest and reset yet, then read on, and we'll add those strings to your bow.
- If you haven't got your ladder against the right wall, then it should become priority number one.

I've spoken earlier about your 'why' and the need to have a bigger reason for doing what you do. At times when you feel like quitting, reflecting on that can be helpful. But what's equally useful is thinking of the old adage: if you want to get out of a hole, the first thing you need to do is stop digging. Or my personal favourite, when it comes to diet, throwing in the towel for the whole day because of one bad meal is the same as getting a flat tyre and then slashing the other three tyres because one went flat. Eating poorly for the whole day because you made one bad food choice is the same as slashing the other three tyres. You wouldn't do it with your car, so don't do it with your food.

2. Reset if you press the f*ck it button

I learnt this strategy from my close friend Trisha Lewis, the best-selling author of the books *Trisha's Transformation: Beat the Bulge and Still Indulge* and *Trisha's 21 Day Reset*. Like most things in these books, this is incredibly obvious and simple but can be difficult to actually apply. If you fall off the track with one meal, you must reset and get back on track with the next meal. If you fall off the track over the weekend, you need to reset and get back on it the following week. If you fall off track for the week, you have to reset and not let it become a month.

Another reason why I'm such an advocate of including foods that you enjoy (to a degree) in your nutritional plan is that doing so prevents you from feeling like you are missing out on something. From my own experience, bingeing on your favourite foods normally happens due to an over-restriction on those foods. When I used to compete in fitness competitions, I would go for six to twelve weeks without eating any chocolate or ice-cream. Then, as soon as the show was over, I would binge on those foods for weeks. Embarrassingly, if you saw me after a show, I'd regularly eaten ice-cream for breakfast and that normally set the tone for the day. I could easily rebound between 5 and 8 kilos in a week after a show. Granted, that was 5 to 8 kilos of weight (water, glycogen, inflammation and so on) and not necessarily all fat, but it shows you how quickly your body can rebound.

The truth is, unless you are trying to step on to the stage for a fitness competition, then this type of restriction is at best, unnecessary and, at worst, completely unsustainable. However, most of us have experienced that restrictive type of eating in some shape or form, either self-imposed or otherwise. We want to lose weight, so we think we can't eat pizza or chocolate and drink beer. That's just not true. Yes, those foods are higher in calories and it's easier to go into a surplus by consuming them, so they're not ideal food choices for a weight-loss goal, but you can still factor them into your plan, like the chocolate bar example cited above.

WHEN TO REST AND WHEN TO PRIORITISE

The key to securing longevity in anything is learning to rest. If you can find a nutritional plan that works for you and you condition yourself to not press the f*ck-it button too often, but learn to reset when you do, it's inevitable that you will hit your weight loss or body compositional goal. But whatever you do, don't quit! If you quit, you go all the way back to the start again. The next time you are struggling with your diet, ask why. Is it too restrictive? Are you not eating enough? Does it not include foods you enjoy? Or do you not have a goal you are working towards? Do you not have a reason for eating a certain way right now?

Get to the root of the problem. Once you do that, you can decide if dieting is or isn't a priority right now. But you're not quitting. You're resting. You're prioritising other things – your job, a new relationship, your studies, whatever. But because you have a nutritional plan versus a diet, it's easier to take the foot off the pedal without stopping completely. If this is your current circumstance, apply a minimum effective dose (MED) to your diet and stick to some basic principles:

- Keep the protein intake moderate.
- Eat plenty of fruits and vegetables.
- Consume healthy fats and complex carbs.
- Don't eat too much sugar.

That alone should keep you feeling fuelled and energised. If your goals change, then you focus more on your diet. It's really that simple. Life isn't about being on a 24/7 diet. It's about finding something that fits into your lifestyle and educating yourself on what works best for you. True, food and nutrition can be a minefield in the beginning, but there are great books, podcasts and various resources out there that can help you learn more about the topic. Alternatively, you can cut that learning curve and hire a coach or join a programme where it's all done for you.

Whatever way you get the knowledge, no one can take it away from you. I'll never forget something one of my mentors asked me at the beginning of my business career. For those of you who are subscribed to my podcast or have been in any of my courses, you know that I like to talk. Thankfully, I'm also keenly aware of my need to shut up when somebody smarter than me is speaking. At the time, she was married to one of my best friends, and one night during dinner, she asked me why I listened to her so attentively when she spoke. This was my answer: 'You run a multimillion-dollar company. You know way more about business than I do. I never want (or wanted) anybody to give me a successful business.

I want to learn how to run one myself.' And that philosophy came from my background in fitness. I always wanted to learn how to get in great shape so that if I ever lost it (through injury, etc.), then I would always be able to get it back again. Educating yourself on nutrition is the same.

Working with coaches, reading books and listening to podcasts gives you the skillset that you can then forever have. It's not easy, but then nothing worth having generally is. It's micro speed and macro patience. In the micro, you focus on the day to day, not pressing the f*ck-it button but resetting if you do. In the macro, you focus on when you should be resting and when you should be prioritising. If you do that, self-sabotage becomes a thing of the past and you finally get out of your own way. This is assuming that education is your primary issue; but what about the emotional element?

EMOTIONAL EATING – WHAT ARE YOUR TRIGGERS?

I'll start by saying if you have a history of disordered eating, deep-rooted or underlying psychological condition or a history of mental health issues, you should seek a counsellor to heal the emotional element of your food relationship. However, if you are somebody who has slipped into a bad habit of using food as a vehicle for state change due to some external or internal issue, then read on.

Most people generally have their strongest food cravings when they are at their weakest point emotionally or when their willpower is at its lowest. It could be after a long day at work, a boss or partner who has been incessantly shouting at them or just general fatigue and tiredness. In a lot of these cases, people can turn to food for comfort – either consciously or unconsciously. My issue was always 'boredom eating'. I found that if I did not have anything to do, I would generally sit in front of the TV and just eat for the evening. As you can probably guess or have experienced yourself, my plate was never loaded with spinach, lettuce and broccoli at this time of the night either. For me, it was always chocolate or ice-cream. This bad habit took me years to break. I tried everything, from doing squats or push-ups during television ad breaks to drinking more water (which just disrupted my sleep as I would have to get up several times in the middle of the night to pee). Eventually, I found that a 6 p.m. cut-off time for eating was the tool that worked most effectively. But what will work best for you? Well, that depends. Before you can put an effective strategy in place, first you need to identify your diet danger zone.

What is your diet danger zone?

We all have one – that time of the day when all the sugary or salted food looks even more tempting than usual. For some, its mid-morning or lunchtime, especially if you skipped breakfast, which I generally do not recommend. For others, it is their commute home from work; you pull up to get petrol and those tasty chocolate bars are just staring at you as you go to pay at the shop counter. If you are like me, it is the evening time. Work is done, the children's homework is finished and it is time to switch off. However, as soon as you hit that point, you are now at the highest risk of falling into the diet danger zone – that time when cravings are at their highest. If this is you, there are a few strategies to help you deal with the diet danger zone.

1. Have a 'cut-off' time for eating.

Pick a time in the evening when you are not going to eat any more food. No meals, no snacks, nothing. If you are eating enough during the day and just picking out of habit or boredom, this is a great strategy to use.

2. Have some herbal tea or coffee.

If you are trying to watch your calorie intake, try making yourself a hot drink after meals. A good piece of advice when eating out or for those lunchtime cravings is to drink a hot coffee, tea or espresso after a meal. Not only will this help you to avoid the temptation of dessert, but coffee in particular can even increase the amount of fullness with the hormone peptide YY. Peptide YY has an appetite-suppressing effect that may help you reduce your calorie intake to support weight loss.[3] The fat loss benefits of coffee and caffeine in general are expanded in the supplement section at the end of the book. Be mindful of caffeine because of its effect on your quality of sleep though. Caffeine can stay in your system for up to 10–11 hours, so if you drink it too late in the day, you might find yourself staring at the bedroom ceiling for the night. An evening alternative is peppermint, camomile or ginger tea – but experiment with what you enjoy the most. If it is later in the day, just make sure it has low or zero levels of caffeine.

3. Eat something low calorie.

The main problem with the diet danger zones is that you are generally not craving green leafy vegetables late in the evening. However, eating something like some fruit and Greek yoghurt could hit the spot nicely. The sugars from the fruit and the protein from the yoghurt should curb most cravings, and as long as it is factored into your daily calories, it is not going to cause excess weight gain.

I will use this to dispel another popular misconception around nutrition – the myth that carbs (or any food) after 6 p.m. will make you fat. This is just not true. Although your body will have some indication of time due to its inbuilt circadian rhythm, saying carbohydrates or any macronutrient/food will make you fat after a certain time of day is just silly. Too many calories are too many calories regardless of what time of the day you eat them. So the next time somebody says to you that carbs or any food after 6 p.m. will make you fat, I want you to reply with the answer I give my clients who need a way to deal with unsolicited advice from friends or family.

Before we see the example, meet Auntie Jane. She is 10 kilos overweight and has been dieting for half her adult life. Once she hears you ate a bowl of porridge before bed, she feels compelled to offer her opinion on it.

Auntie Jane: 'Oh you shouldn't eat carbs after 6 p.m. – that will all turn to fat.'
You: 'Oh really, that's interesting Auntie Jane. Did you know that all money out of an ATM is free after 6 p.m. too?'
Auntie Jane: 'Huh, no it's not. That's silly!'
You: 'Exactly …'

Although generally well-meaning, most advice from non-experts should be taken with a grain of salt. Auntie Jane, a neighbour or your best friend might be the nicest and sweetest person on the planet, but if they are 10 kilos overweight and have been dieting half their adult life, they are probably not the best people to take dietary advice from. If you are wondering who you should take advice from in a non-professional setting, you can filter out 99 per cent of opinions with this one question: would I switch position with the person offering me the advice? If the answer is 'no', then you thank them for their opinion, you disregard it and move on. If the answer is 'yes', then you can think about it more deeply. Of course, this does not apply to professionals, as they have more context on your particular issue, background or situation; but it will help you navigate through the noise of friends, family and work colleagues.

4. Make sure you are eating enough during the day.

Have you ever started a new diet that drastically reduces the amount of food that you eat? It might be a self-inflicted skipping of breakfast mixed with a salad at lunchtime or it might be a new juice, bar or smoothie plan. Either way, you are not eating a lot of food. What normally happens that evening when you get home? You are famished! You probably feel like you could eat everything in sight. Now, do you think your cravings are coming from some emotional issue or did you just starve yourself and that is why you feel this way? It is most likely the latter. This is not an emotional issue, it is an educational one. If this has happened to you on more than one occasion, then I recommend you read (or re-read) Part One of this book in its entirety.

Are there other triggers?

Major life events or, more commonly, the hassles of daily life referred to earlier, can trigger negative emotions that lead to emotional eating and disrupt your weight and fat loss efforts. These triggers might include:

- Relationship conflicts
- Work or other stressors
- Fatigue
- Financial pressures
- Health problems

Truthfully, the list goes on and on. Although some people eat less in the face of strong emotions, as cortisol (the stress hormone) can suppress appetite, others can turn to impulsive or binge eating, quickly consuming whatever is convenient without enjoyment. In fact, I have had clients whose emotions had become so connected to their eating habits that they automatically reached for a 'treat' whenever they were angry or stressed without thinking about what they were doing. Identifying the triggers and then creating an alternative or supportive habit can be the best practice here. I have several case studies around this with clients, but there are so many personal factors to consider that each would be a chapter in itself. However, here is an example of what I did in my own life that summarises a similar approach to the one that I took with my clients.

The year is 2012. At the time, I was working full time as a primary school teacher in West London and had picked up quite a few bad habits. I would come home after work every day, sit in the same chair, watch the same game show and have two or three chocolate bars as I relaxed in front of the TV. I was starting to lose my shape and my energy levels plummeted. I had created a bad habit.

The author of *The Power of Habit*, Charles Duhigg, talks about the 'cue – routine – reward' system of habits. In order to change a habit, you need to change one of the components of this system. The cue is the actual situation or 'trigger' – for me, the cue was coming home every day after work. The routine is what you do next, i.e. getting two or three bars from the cupboard and sitting in the same seat watching the same show. And the reward is serotonin release, the 'happy hormone' your brain releases from the chocolate.

As soon as I realised this was affecting me negatively, I put plans in place to change one of the components. For me, the cue of coming home from work was always going to be the same, so I changed the routine. Instead of reaching for chocolate bars in the cupboard, I left a pre-packed gym bag beside the front door. I would come home (cue), pick up my gym bag (new routine) and the reward came via the serotonin release from exercise. Becoming self-aware of your negative behaviour, patterns and habits is not always that easy to recognise, but once you do, you can make a conscious effort to change it. Another useful tool if you find that your emotional situations drive you towards food is to practise mindful eating.

Mindful eating

This way of eating is about becoming mindful of the food you are eating. Practising mindful eating can help you become more aware of what you are eating, how much you're eating and why you are eating it. This means turning your full attention to the process of choosing, preparing and eating your food, whether that be meals, snacks or drinks.

1. Remove distractions.

The first step to mindful eating is to remove distractions at mealtimes. If you are preoccupied with your surroundings, such as the TV, your mobile phone, driving or work, it is difficult to focus on the process of eating properly. This often leads us to eating more than what our body needs, or eating past the point of fullness. Ideally, try to eat at a table away from your workspace and minimise other distractions. Eating in the company of others is a great way to spend mealtimes.

2. Slow down.

The next step is to take time to eat your meal. Often, we eat food on the go or in a hurry while focusing on something else. The '20, 20, 20' strategy is a helpful tool to increase mindfulness around food and eating. At each meal:

- Chew your food for 20 seconds.
- Put your fork down for 20 seconds between mouthfuls.
- Take 20 minutes to eat your meal.

Concentrate entirely on your food, and even if you feel your mind wandering, carry on. You will likely find that you need to eat less as you become more in tune with your body's hunger signals and more aware of what you are eating.

To listen to my podcast with nutritionist Isa Robinson on Food Addiction, Managing Disordered Eating and the Problem with Diet Culture, go to *www.briankeanefitness.com/the-keane-edge/ bonuses*

How do you get back on track?

When negative emotions threaten to trigger emotional eating, you can take steps to control cravings. Try these tips:

- **Keep a food diary.** Write down what you eat, how much you eat, when you eat, how you are feeling when you eat and how hungry you are. Over time, you might see patterns that reveal the connection between mood and food.

- **Stress management.** If stress contributes to your emotional eating, try a stress management technique such as yoga, meditation or deep breathing. I'm a big a fan of hot Epsom salt baths and/or cold showers, but that is only if you like things a bit more extreme.

- **Check in with your hunger.** Is your hunger physical or emotional? If you ate just a few hours ago and do not have a rumbling stomach, you are probably not hungry. Give the craving time to pass. See the physical vs emotional list at the end of this chapter for more on this.

- **Get support.** You are more likely to give in to emotional eating if you lack a good support network. Lean on family and friends or consider joining a support group or programme.

- **Fight boredom.** Instead of snacking when you are not hungry, distract yourself and substitute a healthier behaviour. Take a walk, watch a movie, play with your kids or pets, listen to music, read or call a friend.

- **Systems over willpower.** Do not keep hard-to-resist comfort foods in your home. And if you feel angry or blue, postpone your trip to the grocery store until you have your emotions in check.

- **Do not deprive yourself.** When trying to lose weight, you might limit calories too much, eat the same foods repeatedly and banish your favourite 'unhealthy' foods. This may just serve to increase your food cravings, especially in response to emotions. Eat satisfying amounts of healthier foods, enjoy an occasional treat and get plenty of variety to help curb cravings.
- **Snack healthily.** If you feel the urge to eat between meals, choose a healthy snack, such as fresh fruit, vegetables with low-fat dip, nuts or unbuttered popcorn. Or try lower-calorie versions of your favourite foods to see if they satisfy your craving.
- **Failure as feedback.** If you have an episode of emotional eating, forgive yourself and start fresh the next day. Try to learn from the experience and plan for how you can prevent it in the future. Focus on the positive changes you are making in your eating habits and give yourself credit for making changes that will lead to better health. In other words, reset and go again.

Finally, it is always worth reminding yourself of the difference between physical and emotional hunger. If you are trying to establish which side you are currently on, run through the table on the next page.

Physical hunger	Emotional hunger
Is gradual	Is sudden
Is open to all different foods	Is usually for a specific food
Based in the stomach	Is based above the neck
Is patient	Is urgent
Occurred out of a physical need	Is paired with an upsetting emotion
Involves deliberate choices and awareness of food	Involves automatic or absent-minded eating
Stops eating when full	Eats until it's uncomfortable
Realises eating is necessary	Feels guilty after eating

Up to this point, we have covered everything you need to do when it comes to your mindset around nutrition. Now let's tackle some of the science, starting with a closer look at macronutrients.

Part Three
Nutrition and Training

Nutrition 101

Macronutrients, or macros for short, are carbohydrates, fats and proteins. So, basically, everything you eat can be broken down into these three macronutrient categories. I'm not going to go into too much detail on them here, as for weight-loss success, the three golden rules are calorie intake, mindset and consistency. With that in mind, here is a straightforward breakdown of each.

CARBOHYDRATES

Whole grains

Whole grains are complex carbohydrates that are not only filling but also nutrient-packed. Here are some of the healthiest options:
- Brown rice
- Wheat (if you're not allergic)
- Barley
- Oats
- Quinoa
- Sweet potatoes

- Baby new potatoes
- Buckwheat

Fruits and vegetables

Although certain fruits have high levels of natural sugar, they're still a healthier substitute than some of our favourite carb-ridden snacks. Here's a sampling of fruits and vegetables that contain complex carbohydrates:

- Potatoes
- Tomatoes
- Onions
- Okra
- Dill pickles
- Carrots
- Yams
- Strawberries
- Peas
- Radishes
- Beans
- Broccoli
- Spinach
- Green beans
- Zucchini
- Apples
- Pears
- Cucumbers
- Asparagus
- Grapefruit
- Prunes

The benefits of complex carbohydrates

Complex carbohydrates – the 'good' type of carb – provide the body some of what it needs to operate at peak performance. Here are a few reasons to choose complex carbohydrates over simple carbohydrates.

- **Fuel.** Complex carbs keep the body fuelled for an extended period of time. This is especially important if you are following any form of intense training programme. Carbs will help fuel and improve recovery from workouts. If you struggle to increase your carb intake due to years of misinformation around them, remember carbs don't make you fat, too many calories make you fat.

- **Digestion.** Complex carbohydrates take longer to digest. This makes them key to fulfilling hunger as well as providing a longer-lasting source of energy. Because complex carbohydrates often have lots of fibre, this bulks up stool, allowing it to move smoothly through the digestive tract. When this occurs, less bloating and gas exist, constipation can be lessened and more toxins are removed from the body.

- **Weight loss.** Yes, the right carbs can actually help you lose weight, not gain weight. Eating complex carbohydrates helps you feel full for a longer period of time. As a result, cravings are lessened and the need to reach for unhealthy snacks between planned meals is diminished. As long as they are within a calorie-controlled plan, you will still lose fat eating carbohydrates.

FATS

Similar to carbohydrates, there are a lot of misconceptions around fats. For example, some nutritionists say saturated fat should be avoided completely, others consider it to be a health staple to balance hormones. Instead of focusing on that, include a decent amount of fats in your plan to help balance hormones, curb hunger pangs and improve brain cognition. Just be aware that high-fat foods tend to be more calorific. For example: 1g of protein or carbohydrate = 4kcal, while 1g of fat = 9kcal. That's not to say you should avoid them – you shouldn't – but be aware that the calorie content is generally higher compared to the other macronutrients.

Monounsaturated fat

Good sources include:
- Olive, canola, peanut and sesame oils
- Avocados
- Olives
- Nuts (almonds, peanuts, macadamia, hazelnuts, pecans, cashews)
- Peanut butter

Polyunsaturated fat

Good sources include:
- Sunflower, sesame and pumpkin seeds
- Flaxseed
- Walnuts
- Tofu

- Fatty fish (salmon, tuna, mackerel, herring, trout, sardines) and fish oil
- Soybean and safflower oil
- Soymilk

Saturated fat

Primary sources include:
- Red meat (beef, lamb, pork)
- Chicken skin
- Whole-fat dairy products (milk, cream, cheese)
- Butter
- Coconut oil

PROTEIN (AMINO ACIDS)

Amino acids are the building blocks of protein. There are over two hundred in total, some toxic and some essential to human life. An essential amino acid is defined as 'one which cannot be synthesised by the animal organism out of materials ordinarily available to cells at a speed commensurate with the demands for normal growth'[4] – simply put, you need to get them from food or supplements.

Twenty-one of the existing amino acids are required for protein synthesis, including repair and growth of lean muscle tissue. If you want to tone up, increase your metabolism or build muscle, hitting your daily protein requirements is a necessity. However, the following amino acids cannot be created by the body:
- Isoleucine
- Leucine

- Valine (these first three are the make-up of the popular sports supplement Branch Chain Amino Acids that is regularly used for recovery in athletes)
- Lysine
- Methionine
- Phenylalanine
- Threonine
- Tryptophan
- Histidine

Complete protein foods have all the essential amino acids our bodies need. Incomplete protein sources are normally plant-based and require food combinations or a varied diet in order to get everything you need from food. If you follow a vegan-based nutritional plan or lifestyle, then this is worth researching further.

Here are some examples of complete protein sources:

- Fish and seafood
- Skinless, white-meat poultry
- Beef (including tenderloin, sirloin, etc.)
- Skim or low-fat milk
- Skim or low-fat yoghurt
- Fat-free or low-fat cheese
- Eggs
- Pork (tenderloin)

In the last section of the book, we will go through a sample meal plan and some recipes. The foods listed above are just to give you an idea of the categories that they fall into. This isn't a 'eat this and not that' book – far from it. For now, we're going to keep it practical and talk about how to navigate popular topics like alcohol consumption and managing the weekend.

TIPS FOR EATING OUT AND ALCOHOL CONSUMPTION

This topic can be a bit of a sticky point for a lot of us. You've seen why your mindset plays such an important role in your weight-loss journey. You're ready to make the nutritional changes that can positively impact your waistline and then BANG! life happens. A wedding, a night out or even a simple evening meal at a restaurant. Suddenly, the temptation to press the f*ck-it button comes back stronger than ever. Before you do that, here are some tips and tricks so you can have the best of all worlds. Eat what you want in the restaurant or have a few drinks and still lose weight!

Banking calories for the weekend

In Part One I spoke about how calories are similar to your finances, and here I'm going to give you another example which will support you the most if you're looking to have nutritional flexibility during weekends.

Meet my friend Josh. Josh works nine to five, Monday to Friday, and likes a good night out during the weekend. The problem is that he easily spends €100 every Saturday night at his favourite restaurant and bar. However, he's also sensible enough to save a little bit every week. Josh earns €500 per week from his job. He spends about €350 on rent, food, travel and miscellaneous things – this includes all his weekly expenditure except his Saturday night out. This leaves him with €150 disposable income every week. Now, Josh can put €50 aside and save it every week while still having his €100 to spend on his favourite thing in the world: his Saturday night out. It won't happen by chance. He needs to be somewhat disciplined during the week in order to not go over his allowance, but by and large, this routine works tremendously well for him. What has this got to do with weight loss? Actually, the situation is nearly identical. You are just replacing money with calories. If you don't want to sacrifice your nights out or weekly meals at your favourite restaurants, then you don't have to. You just need to factor them into your calorie budget for the week. For example, if you want to have 1,000kcal from beer, wine and/or your favourite meal, then you cut back or 'bank' some of your calories earlier in the week. This doesn't have to be super-complicated either. If you know you have a weekend of partying ahead of you, you could drop 100–200kcal from your food consumption for Monday to Friday. You can do this by having slightly smaller dinner portions, cutting back on snacks and so on – nothing drastic though.

Then, you can use those 'banked' calories during the weekend. As we know by now, to lose weight, you need to be in an overall caloric deficit. Even if you had a controlled 'blow out' on a Saturday night and are still in a deficit come the end of the week, you'll continue to reduce body fat. The key is to be conscious of how many calories you are actually consuming, or at least to have a general idea. Pressing the f*ck-it button or having a Last Supper every weekend isn't helpful either, but 'banking' of calories can work great if you're someone who likes the best of all worlds and wants weekend flexibility with your nutrition.

The importance of 'cheat' or 'free' meals

First, another 250-kilo gorilla in the room needs to be addressed. I hate the term 'cheat' meal. For me, it goes against my entire philosophy of not separating food into 'good' and 'bad' categories.

Remember, food has no morals. A 'cheat' meal can make you feel like you've done something wrong and it's generally not the most supportive association to have with food.

I like to refer to it as a 'free' meal. This is a food choice that isn't necessarily on your plan; it's probably high in calories and devoid of nutrients, but it's a food or meal choice that you love! Think ice-cream, chocolate, biscuits, cakes, takeaways. Similar to 'banking' calories above, a free meal is also structured. It's planned; every Friday or Saturday night, you have your weekly 'free' meal. Not only is there a great psychological benefit to free meals, but they also serve a metabolic function as well.

At this stage, you're hopefully no longer separating food into good and bad categories, but try to remember this tip if you're someone who still struggles with guilt or shame around eating 'bad' food. A weekly free meal, where you go over your calorie intake for the day, has been proven to boost your metabolism and can potentially ward off any feelings of deprivation, improving not only your ability to lose weight but also your ability to stick to your diet plan.[5]

One way free meals can boost your metabolism is by increasing levels of leptins, the 'anti-starvation' hormone responsible for sending hunger messages to the brain. Throwing a free meal into the mix tricks your system into thinking that food is plentiful and that it's okay to burn through fat stores. Planning is the key when it comes to free meals. I recommend scheduling it for a time when you're most likely to be craving fatty foods, such as on a weekend or a special occasion. This way, you can fit it around your calorie intake that week or day, and it's great to have something to look forward to, giving you that extra motivation to do well during the week. This also allows you to choose a 'free meal' you'll really enjoy. However, it's important not to press the f*ck-it button and let your free meals turn into free day(s). We've discussed this more in the chapter on self-sabotage; so, if you find your free meals turning into free days or free weeks, refer to that section again.

As a side note, I'd advise that you don't weigh yourself for at least two to three days after your free meal. As long as you are still in an overall calorie deficit, you should still make progress even if the scale number increases. Remember, for every gram of carbohydrate you consume, your body holds between 2–3 grams of water. Plan for extra water consumption on the day after your free meal in order to balance this back out. If you still struggle to wrap your head around the sudden weight gain, refer back to Part One and the difference between losing weight and losing body fat.

How to fit in alcohol

This is a tricky one. Although alcohol has what are called 'empty calories', i.e. calories with no real nutritional value or benefit, not all alcoholic drinks are created equal when it comes to their caloric value.

My recommendation is that you decide on whether you want to include alcohol in your plan or not. If you want to look your best for an occasion in the future, and really want to reduce body fat, then I'd recommend abstaining from the empty calories of alcohol until that date. However, if you're looking for a more balanced approach whereby you can include alcohol and not have it negatively affect your waistline, then look at the calories of your drink of choice. For example, look at this comparison:

Three pints of beer: 600–900kcal
Three glasses of white wine: 246kcal
Three glasses of vodka and diet mixer: 192kcal

It's worth adding that alcohol can negatively impact your progress in a few other ways too. As alcohol is metabolised by the liver and thus drastically affects your blood sugar balance, particularly when consumed on an empty stomach, it can lead to a sense of increased hunger, which can potentially lead to overeating. If you've ever devoured a full pizza or curry cheese chips after a night out, you'll know exactly what I'm talking about here. True, the lack of inhibitions that come with alcohol don't help here either, but the physiological blood sugar issues make it a real 'one-two knockout punch'.

However, in line with my philosophy throughout this book, if you enjoy it, one or two glasses of wine or beer won't impact the results too drastically. A full bottle of wine or 10 beers is a different story now. The same goes for your weekly night out. If you have six glasses of vodka and a diet mixer, that's only about 400kcal; just make sure it doesn't lead to poor food choices that night or the dreaded comfort food bang-up fry the following day.

THE SEVEN DEADLY DIET SINS

Do you think you're doing everything right, yet don't see any results? In 99 per cent of cases, I normally find one or several of the issues below are the culprit. I call them 'the Seven Deadly Diet Sins'. As you know by now, I don't like the word 'diet', but 'the Seven Deadly Nutrition Sins' just doesn't have the same ring to it.

One of my favourite quotes is by the Nobel Prize winner, physicist Richard Feynman, who said: 'You must not fool yourself – and you are the easiest person to fool', and the Seven Deadly Diet Sins are based on this principle. These are the areas of nutrition you need to keep a close eye on – your 'blind spots' – things you may not even be aware you are doing, which are consciously or subconsciously hindering your weight-loss goal.

Time and time again, I have worked with people who are convinced they are doing all the right things when it comes to lowering body fat; however, once we go through the list below, there is always at least that one thing that is obstructing their progress. The extreme examples of why you cannot lose weight are normally pretty self-evident: if you eat several Chinese takeaways every week or drink two litres of full-sugar soda every day, it is pretty obvious where the change needs to occur. But what if you don't do these things? The Seven Deadly Diet Sins are things that people forget to do or are unaware they are doing (either consciously or subconsciously), which leads to them consuming extra calories throughout the day. I am aware that 'thou shalt not' is from the biblical 10 commandments; but, similar to using the word 'diet' for this section, I have taken some creative liberty with how I portray this essential information.

1. Thou shalt not fool thyself with treats

Do you sit down every night with a biscuit and a cup of tea? You have eaten well all day, hit your daily step count or went to the gym, and this is your 'treat time'. One biscuit would not set you back, right? About 40–100kcal, depending on the biscuit, is factored into your plan and still keeps you in the calorie deficit plan for the day. Great. Enjoy. But is it really only *one* biscuit that you are eating, or did you have two or three? Perhaps you allowed yourself two or three but have actually had five or six instead. Again, I am not asking you not to enjoy your favourite foods, far from it, but too many calories is too many calories. Also, biscuits, chocolates and savoury or sweet foods are very easy to overeat. If you are planning on having two biscuits every evening, then eat two biscuits and put the packet away; or, you can eat the entire packet if you want to, just make sure you realign your expectations. If you have eaten half a packet or a full packet of biscuits, then it is unlikely that your body fat is going to reduce in the coming days. The choice is yours though. As long as you are not fooling yourself, I am okay with whatever choice you make.

2. Thou shalt not pick food off thy kid's plate (or thy partner's plate or anyone else's plate)

I cannot really talk in this matter as I am terrible for picking oven-baked chips off my daughter's plate. My solution to this is to make sure I have my own food in front of me when she is eating. Again, do not be fooled by '*the calories on my plate are the only calories that count*' – your body does not care if they are from your plate, your child's plate or from the moon. Too many calories are too many calories.

3. Thou shalt not forget to count alcoholic calories

As discussed above, counting alcoholic calories is obvious to most of us. However, the amount normally surprises people; therefore, use the alcohol calorie chart as a reference to make choices that align with your goals.

4. Thou shalt not disregard that portion size matters (extra food = extra calories, regardless of how healthy or 'clean' it is)

I have already discussed the fallacy of clean eating earlier in the book and how too many calories are too many calories, whether it is from takeaway and chocolate or chicken and broccoli; so, your portion size matters. Being aware of this is normally enough for most people; however, you can try this simple food swap alternative if you think it will support you. Instead of loading up on complex carbs such as rice and potatoes at lunch or dinner time, keep those portion sizes to the palm of your hand and then load up on veggies to keep the calorie count lower. Not only will the fibre keep you feeling fuller for longer but the micronutrient profile of vegetables, green leafy ones in particular, are great for overall health and energy levels.

5. Thou shalt not over-restrict then binge (the 'but I've eaten well all week' fallacy)

Yup, we are back here again. You can have calorie deficit meals Monday to Friday and then binge with too many calories at the weekend. This will still lead to fat gain if it equates to an overall calorie surplus at the end of the week. Not only does this damage and strain your relationship with food but it is also a terrible strategy for long-term weight loss.

6. Thou shalt not have unhealthy snacks alongside healthy meals

Another problem I encounter a lot is a person who eats a high-quality breakfast, lunch and dinner, but then snacks on rubbish throughout the day. Again, this one is relatively easy to recognise, but it is normally wrapped up in the story of 'I eat well most of the time' – usually followed by '… but I eat a lot of rubbish as well'. Again, I am not asking you to avoid these foods; but if you are snacking on chocolates, packets of crisps and biscuits in between meals, you either need to reduce your calorie intake elsewhere (portion size at major meals) or switch up some of your snacks. Generally, switching out sweets for fruit or savoury food for nuts can be a nice transition point for most.

7. Thou shalt not forget why thou are doing it in the first place

The other six sins feed into this one. Truth be told, the 'commandments' are only difficult to follow if you are wilfully blind to them for whatever reason (see the emotional eating section earlier in the book) or you do not know why you are bothering in the first place. Of course, picking chips off your partner's plate or grabbing a chocolate bar at lunchtime is going to be tempting if you have no reason not to do it. Make sure you are clear on your reason for wanting to reduce body fat, lose weight or look better; that is your anchor for avoiding the other six sins.

If you see yourself in any of the examples above, just be aware of it going forward. You do not have to make any drastic changes, but bring some awareness to your actions and when or if you decide to change that pattern of behaviour, you can use some of the other tools in this book to do so. Awareness is always the first step towards change.

HOW TO BREAK THROUGH A WEIGHT-LOSS PLATEAU

In the course of my 10-plus years working in the fitness industry, 99 per cent of 'weight-loss plateaus' I've encountered were down to the same causes. One was due to tracking the wrong metric, i.e. weight loss, which fluctuates daily, vs fat loss, which doesn't. The other was a misalignment of expectation due to initial progress, starter momentum or 'beginner gains', where your expectations are too high due to initial progress from switching something in your nutrition, exercise regimen or lifestyle in general. This normally comes in the form of a dramatic weight drop in week one, looser-fitting clothing in weeks two and three or a dramatic photo change in week six. Then tangible progress slows down from week six onwards.

Progress isn't always in an upward momentum. If they're maintaining their calorie deficit, most people will continue to lower body fat over time, but the *speed* of that progress could slow down as your body becomes more accustomed to what you're doing. Of course, there are the exceptions to this rule, the 1 per cent of people who are genuinely hitting a fat-loss plateau due to some hormonal disruption – a thyroid issue, excessive cortisol or a problem with oestrogen or testosterone – However, for most of us, if you were to rigorously test your body fat levels each week in a laboratory or through a DXA scanner, you would see that your fat levels *are* reducing, just at a slower rate than the previous six weeks.

With that knowledge, the power is back in your hands and you have a choice to make. You can continue to cultivate the patience needed to continue your progress over time or you can make more dramatic changes to push past this 'speed of progress plateau'. If patience is your strategy, then your mindset remains your primary focus. If speeding up your progress is the goal, then try one or all of the techniques below to break the weight-loss plateau.

Carb cycling

At this stage, you understand how important your calorie intake is on a weight-loss journey, but that doesn't mean you can't adjust your macronutrients in order to speed up progress. Carbohydrates are the focus of this tactic, most notably, cycling your carbohydrate intake day to day. Carb cycling is effectively when you cycle (reduce or increase) your carbohydrate intake on different days. Here's a simple breakdown:

- Low carb on rest days.
- Moderate carb on training days (gym or HIIT training).
- High carb the day before or day of intense training sessions (a weekly leg workout or a particularly difficult HIIT session, for example).

The numbers vary greatly from person to person, and very much depend on your training programme, your metabolism and your lifestyle in general. Just to give you a range, I've had some of my clients go with 50g of carbs of low days, 150g on moderate and 300g on high days, while others have used 200g on low days, 400g on moderate days and 800g on high days.

Individual requirements will be different, but for simplicity, I'm going to use 100g for low days, 200g for moderate and 300g for high days as the numbers going forward. Of course, your individual requirements will be different but the simple 100g, 200g and 300g should help to illustrate how carb cycling works.

Carb cycling with complex carbs

Carbohydrates are traditionally classified according to their chemical structure. The most simplistic method divides them into two categories: simple (sugars) and complex (starches and fibres). These terms simply refer to the number of sugar units in the molecule. Simple carbohydrates are very small molecules consisting of one or two sugar units. They comprise monosaccharides (one sugar unit); glucose (dextrose, which is in a lot of sports performance drinks); fructose (fruit sugar) and galactose (found in milk); and the disaccharides (two sugar units): sucrose (normal table sugar, which is a mixture of glucose and fructose) and lactose (milk sugar, which is a mixture of glucose and galactose). Lactose intolerance is an inability to break down the sugar lactose, and if you can't process lactose there are great alternatives on the market – coconut milk or yoghurt or almond-based alternatives work great for most people.

Complex carbohydrates are much larger molecules, consisting of between 10 and several thousand sugar units (mostly glucose) joined together. They include the starches, amylose and amylopectin, and the non-starch polysaccharides (dietary fibre) such as cellulose, pectin and hemicellulose.

Many foods contain a mixture of both simple and complex carbohydrates, making the traditional classification of food into 'simple' and 'complex' very confusing. The 'majority rules' tend to apply here too. If a food is mostly made up of complex carbs (oats, sweet potato, brown rice, etc.), we call it a complex carb; if it's mostly made up of simple sugars (cakes, biscuits, etc.), we normally call it a simple sugar.

There's a time and place for different types of carbohydrates and an 80:20 rule works very well here. I recommend carb cycling with 80 per cent of your intake from complex carbohydrates and 20 per cent from simple sugars. They can come in the form of a chocolate or protein bar during the day to support adherence, or holding off for a free meal at the weekend. This varies from person to person but tends to work well for most. Although it's tempting to think that simple carbohydrates, due to their smaller molecular size, are absorbed more quickly than complex carbohydrates, and produce a rapid rise in blood sugar, it's not always the case. For example, many starchy foods (complex carbohydrates), such as white potatoes and white bread are digested and absorbed very quickly and give a rapid rise in blood sugar. With the exception of right before, during or after training, spiking your blood sugar is normally best avoided.

Another misleading food is an apple (that contains simple carbohydrates): although it's a fruit, it produces a small and prolonged rise in blood sugar, despite being high in simple carbohydrates. Apples contain a type of fibre called pectin, which is found between the cell walls of plants and is classified as soluble fibre. This type of fibre has been shown to slow down digestion by attracting water and forming a gel which ultimately helps you feel fuller for longer and gives you a steadier release of energy. This makes it a great snack during the day, or as an energy hit before a workout.

To confuse things even more, most – but not all – fruits spike blood sugars, as do potatoes and bread – but not sweet potato or wholegrain bread. What's more important as far as weight loss is concerned is how rapidly the carbohydrate is absorbed from the small intestine into your bloodstream. The faster this transfer, the more rapidly the carbohydrate can be taken up by muscle cells and make a difference to your training, performance and recovery. The system that generally helps people to wrap their heads around this is the glycaemic index.

The glycaemic index

To describe more accurately the effect different foods have on your blood sugar levels, scientists developed the glycaemic index (GI). Simply put, this index, which goes from 0 to 100, indicates how quickly a food raises blood sugar levels. Glucose is rated at 100, and the closer to 100 a food is rated; the more it affects blood sugar levels.

In her book *The Complete Guide to Sports Nutrition,* Anita Bean explains using an example of a baked potato. For example, to test baked potatoes, you would eat 250g of potatoes, which contain 50g of carbohydrate. Over the next two hours, a sample of blood is taken every 15 minutes and the blood sugar measured. The blood sugar is plotted on a graph and the area under the curve calculated. Your response to the test food (e.g. potatoes) is compared with your blood sugar response to 50g of glucose (the reference food). The GI is given as a percentage, which is calculated by dividing the area under the curve after you've eaten potatoes by the area under the curve after you've eaten the glucose. So, the GI of baked potatoes is 85, which means that eating a baked potato produces a rise in blood sugar which is 85 per cent as great as that produced after eating an equivalent amount of glucose.

The GI of more than 600 foods is known, and although you definitely don't need to know all 600, it helps to have an idea of a few of the low-GI, slow-digesting complex carbs so you can factor your favourite ones into your plan. I've found that my clients tend to find it easier to classify foods as high GI (60–100), medium GI (40–59) and low GI (less than 40).

- Low-GI complex carbohydrates: oats, quinoa, brown rice, wholewheat pasta, green vegetables, certain fruits, raw carrots, lentils
- Medium GI: basmati rice, wholegrain bread, sweetcorn, bananas, raw pineapple, raisins, oat breakfast cereals, multi-grain, oat bran or rye bread
- High GI: dextrose, glucose, watermelon, white bread, white pasta, white potatoes, full-sugar soda, most breakfast cereals and cereal bars

This isn't to say that there aren't more or better options; these are just some of the popular food options that are available in most places.

It's worth noting that the speed at which blood sugar levels can rise is also dependent on the food combinations in a meal. For example, having a simple sugar with a fat source will slow down the speed at which it raises blood sugar. This won't matter too much if you are eating mostly low or medium GI and slowly digesting carbs – having a fat source or protein source with it may just slow it down further and shouldn't have any negative effect on your blood sugar levels. On top of keeping your blood sugar levels stable so you're not on a rollercoaster of energy all day, the fibre in these foods tend to keep you feeling fuller for longer, which can work great for adherence on a fat loss plan.

Slow- or fast-digesting carbs before training?

Whether to eat high-GI or low-GI food before training has long been a controversial area. Some scientific studies and anecdotal evidence swear by having simple sugars before training; others swear by having complex carbs before training. Again, the truth is probably somewhere in the middle. Some people work better with fast carbohydrates before training, others perform better with slow carbohydrates before training; others do well with a combination of both. I recommend experimenting and seeing what works best for you to push past a weight-loss plateau. If you find that your workout is greatly enhanced by consuming some simple sugars before your workouts and you're maintaining an overall caloric deficit, then this might be the perfect thing that pushes you past your plateau. Increased exercise intensity generally equates towards more calories burnt. More calories burnt generally equals pushing past on a fat-loss plateau. Which brings me to my next point – exercising to push past a weight-loss plateau.

Mixing up your workouts

There are two schools of thought when it comes to mixing up your workouts. One is the 'muscle confusion principle', where you continually switch up your workout's routines in order to 'keep your body guessing', and to some degree, this may be true. Doing something new tends to require extra effort on the part of your body and can potentially result in an increase in metabolism. If you are used to running, for example, lifting weights will likely challenge your body in a different way and can potentially have a positive effect on metabolism. Ditto for a weightlifter who starts to run. The evidence on this is largely anecdotal at this point; but the behavioural change element and keeping motivation high due to switching things up has been known by professional trainers for decades. If you're finding your workout tedious and boring, then it might be time to try something new. For more on this, check out the training chapter.

The second school of thought is 'primary goal theory', where you make sure your training programme is in perfect alignment with your goal and changing it up regularly is less important than making sure the programme is correct in the first place. This has obvious benefits too. If you're training for a marathon, your programme should include running and maybe some gym-supported assistive work too. If you want to be a bodybuilder, running in your programme becomes less important but your exercise choice, reps, sets and rest that work within hypertrophy – muscle building – come to the forefront.

Of course, like most things, the truth is probably a combination of both. Make sure you are doing a workout programme that's in alignment with your specific goals; but mix it up regularly, every six weeks or so, to ensure you don't get bored and can continue to progress. That brings me on to the final tip for breaking through a weight-loss plateau, setting a new goal for yourself.

Setting a new goal

Changing up your goal can not only work wonders for motivation, it can support a weight-loss goal too. If you have been doing HIIT workouts for the past six weeks and feel you are starting to plateau a bit, maybe it's time to sign up to a couch to 5 K run, a 10 K fun run or a half marathon. The new goal focus can get you excited about training again, and the switch from HIIT to more of a running-based programme can potentially have a positive metabolic impact too. The same works in reverse; if jogging or running is your primary source of exercise, maybe it's time to switch to a HIIT routine or weight workouts. Maybe your new goal consists of hitting a personal best on a squat or deadlift, it really doesn't matter; as long as you are excited about what you are doing or you're enjoying the process of your exercise choice, once the workout supports your end goal of weight loss, then that's what matters. So experiment, find what you enjoy and set new goals regularly to push past plateaus.

WHAT TO AVOID, MINIMISE OR CONSUME TO YOUR HEART'S CONTENT

Most people would love to have a list of foods, drinks and ingredients to avoid, or consume at will, in the course of a weight-loss programme. However, everything I've listed here has pros and cons and your dietary history, genetic makeup, gut microbiome or even lifestyle choices up to this point will all influence how your body is going to respond, either positively, negatively or neutrally. So I'm going to lay out the facts for you and then you can make an informed decision on whether or not to include them in your nutritional plan. I'll also explain what I do personally in each scenario, and the reasons for my choices, as this may help you to navigate on whether their inclusion or exclusion should be your primary focus.

Gluten: the facts

Let's start with the monster under the bed: gluten. I've never seen a family of proteins – gluten being a family of proteins found in grains, including wheat, rye, spelt and barley – that has been demonised by so many. I'll admit at the outset that I myself have not eaten gluten in nearly two decades. I had a whole host of digestive, hormonal and mental health issues in my teenage years, all of which I've since addressed; but the experience left a deep imprint. One of the dietary interventions for me at the time was the removal of gluten from my daily eating plan. I had and have what is now commonly referred to as non-coeliac gluten sensitivity. It means that gluten makes me feel sick, but it's not potentially fatal if I continue to eat it. If you have coeliac disease or, like me, non-coeliac gluten sensitivity, i.e. you get serious stomach distress, a distended stomach and diarrhoea if you eat it, then you should avoid it. Simple as that. If you don't have those issues, that is where it gets interesting.

Over the past decade, gluten has acquired a bad reputation. Everyone, regardless of expertise, seems to have an opinion, with social media influencers, celebrities and even doctors labelling gluten as unhealthy, unnecessary and potentially dangerous. Wait, did he say doctors? Unfortunately, I did. Let's digress for a moment as this is pretty important. Just to clarify, I'm not questioning the methods of doctors or Western medicine in general; I'm very grateful for the scientific discoveries made in this area over the past century. But that still doesn't change the fact that most doctors get between 10 and 25 hours of nutritional training over their entire time spent in medical school. Some nutritional audiobooks are longer than that.

I have a story from my time working as a 1:1 personal trainer that summarises this perfectly. I had been working with one of my female clients for about four months. She was 24 at the time – fit, young and healthy. After hitting her weight-loss target, she wanted to take a break from her nutrition and training for a few weeks. We hadn't designed a lifestyle plan at the time, as I was working more as a transformation coach back then. Anyways, she pulled me aside after we had our first training session after a month's break. She told me she was having some issues with her energy levels and thought that her blood sugar levels were too low. For context, she had gone from eating a relatively clean caloric deficit to eating whatever she wanted. She was concerned about her energy levels, so she went to her local doctor to get her blood work done. Everything came back fine, and when she asked about her energy issues, he said it was probably down to low blood sugar. Nothing too astray so far. Then came the kicker. When she asked what she should do, he said, and I quote, 'anytime you feel your blood sugar levels dropping or your energy is low, just have some white bread and jam, that should boost your energy quickly.' Now, credit where credit is due, I have to commend him for not prescribing a random drug or medicine that she didn't need, but as a nutritionist, this advice is nearly as bad as it could possibly be. For the record, the general recommendation for balancing your blood sugar level is normally down to consuming a combination of complex carbohydrates with adequate fibre, some healthy fats and some protein. It's generally recommended that you limit refined sugar or anything that spikes your blood glucose levels too high during this time (sorry, white bread and jam, that's you out my friend).

The advice was nearly the polar opposite to what most qualified nutritionists or registered dietitians will tell you. Now I shouldn't blame the doctor, he's not a nutritionist or a dietitian. I wouldn't expect to go to my car mechanic and get a killer haircut and I wouldn't go to my barber to fix the engine in my car. But save the dietary questions for qualified nutritionists or registered dietitians, or if you do want to get advice from your doctor, find out if they have nutritional knowledge – there are some GPs out there who merge Western medicine with a functional nutritional approach while looking at everything as a whole. Dr Rupy Aujla (aka The Doctor's Kitchen) or Dr Hazel Wallace (aka The Food Medic) are two who I highly recommend following for nutritional advice that merges the best of Western medicine and nutrition.

To listen to my podcast with The Doctor's Kitchen or The Food Medic, go to *www.briankeanefitness.com/the-keane-edge /bonuses*

Now, back to gluten. The wealth of misinformation circulating about gluten and the dearth of good advice on nutrition from professionals has led to the rise in popularity of gluten-free and low-gluten diets. Gluten is one of the most consumed proteins in the world. It's everywhere – in bread, pasta, pastries and biscuits as well as less obvious sources such as beer, soy sauce and my daughter's favourite, gravy.

A very small minority (less than 1 per cent of the population) has no choice but to avoid gluten completely: those who have been medically diagnosed with coeliac disease, or even more rarely, a wheat allergy. Coeliac disease is a proven allergy to gluten; it is an autoimmune disease where your own immune system attacks your tissues when you eat gluten. One of my school friends, Liam, a medically diagnosed coeliac, couldn't even eat the smallest morsel of gluten or he would experience a catalogue of debilitating and unpleasant symptoms. For him, the only way to manage his symptoms was with a gluten-free diet. Knowing what I know now, the damage to his gut would be clearly visible under a microscope, which is why suspected patients will have a tiny piece of their small intestine tested as part of the diagnostic process. This is what happened to me when I was tested for coeliac disease at the age of 15. Crucially, albeit agonisingly as I reflect, I had to eat gluten every day for six weeks prior to the medical test to ensure accurate results. Although it yielded a negative result, I still lost several kilos in the weeks preceding it and was sleeping for more than 13 hours every day! Non-coeliac gluten sensitivity is no joke. If you're regularly consuming a food that your body isn't capable of digesting efficiently, then that's going to lead to a whole host of potential problems.

Despite the current popularity of gluten-free diets and their obvious supportive nature towards calorie reduction by avoiding biscuits, pizza crust and cakes, there is no good evidence that avoiding wheat is good for you. It really depends on what you replace the eliminated food with. If you've replaced biscuits with rice, corn cakes or, better yet, fruit and vegetables, you're probably going to save on calories, and that can support your weight-loss goal. If you replace biscuits with gluten-free biscuits that have the same or higher sugar or calorie content, then nothing will be lighter except for your wallet; gluten-free alternatives can be pretty damn expensive.

Again, if you want to experiment with the removal of gluten from your diet, then by all means try it. Just don't think that going gluten free is going to address your weight problem, simply because 'gluten is bad' or more inaccurately 'gluten makes you fat'. It's worth being aware of the nutritional drawbacks of a gluten-free diet too. Gluten-free products are typically low in vitamin B12, folate, zinc, magnesium, selenium and calcium. This won't be an issue if you're following a well-rounded, nutritionally dense plan, but if you're subbing gluten foods for their non-gluten alternatives, it could be.

Another thing to consider is that commercially produced gluten-free products are often highly refined and calorie dense due to the complex ingredient substitutions required to get close to the textural properties that gluten provides. Normal gluten, which means 'glue' in Latin, is formed when water is mixed with flour, and it gives dough its characteristic texture, elasticity and shape. A recent study[6] found that gluten-free pasta caused consistently higher blood glucose peaks compared with the original wheat varieties. This may be because a range of highly refined carbohydrate products are used to mimic the texture of wheat, meaning that the sugars are quickly released.

As I said, the choice is yours. If you think you will be more likely to adhere to your nutritional plan by completely eliminating gluten, then remove it. Equally, if you think you will be more likely to adhere to your nutritional plan by including your favourite gluten-rich foods, then include them. But make the decision from an informed perspective and not because some randomer on the internet told you to.

Dairy: the facts

There are generally two opposing schools of thought when it comes to dairy, and my goodness, are they opposing. One school will cite the historical inclusion of dairy as far back as the agricultural revolution and shout from the rooftops about the calcium content and benefits to bone health. The other side will lambast you for drinking milk because you're a human being and not a baby calf, therefore arguing that its highly unnatural for you to ingest.

As you'll see, the truth is in the middle again. If you have a dairy allergy or lactose intolerance and milk or other dairy products makes you feel sick, ill or digestively uncomfortable, then you should avoid them. If you have no issues with the ingestion of dairy – no digestive issues, no inflammatory response, such as a runny nose – then include it in your plan. Again, there's probably an element of danger in the dose: milk is generally paired with a morning breakfast cereal and this is not a great way to start your day in regard to high-quality nutrition. Traditional breakfast cereals, although fortified with vitamins, most of which have poor absorption due to the low bioavailability, are generally not considered an ideal breakfast option. But context is key. If you are having a bowl of cereal every morning, one could argue that as long as the rest of your day is full of nutrient-dense food choices and it's within your calorie intake for the day, it should be perfectly fine. Maybe this is the case but I've been a long-term subscriber of making good supportive foods choices in your opening meal and building on that throughout the day. Will a small drop of milk in your coffee or tea impact your weight-loss goals? Very unlikely. Will a glass or two a day add inches to your waistline? Again, if you have no issue digesting it and it's within your calorie allowance for the day, the answer is also no.

Personally I haven't drunk milk since I was 16 years of age. I had a history of sinus issues in my teenage years and one of the categories recommended to eliminate was dairy (gluten was the other). Since then, any time I consume too much dairy, my nose gets all blocked up and I get a little bit of mental fog. There are some studies[7] to suggest that both milk and gluten can cause mental fog, but there are so many gut microbiome and hereditary genetic variabilities to consider that saying everyone should avoid them would not only be a poor recommendation, but also bad science.

So if you have no issue with dairy and you enjoy dairy products, include them. If, like me, you have issues with these foods, avoid or minimise them. It really is as simple as that.

Sugar: the facts

Also known as sucrose, sugar is a simple disaccharide consisting of glucose and fructose, available in the forms of white sugar, brown sugar, malt, maple syrup, honey and a variety of syrups from gains and roots. Being a fast energy-releasing substance, sugar can have a time and a place in a nutritional plan; a lot of marathon runners will use simple sugars on their journey to completing the 26.2-mile race, for example. But context matters. Too much sugar and low activity levels can lead to Type 2 diabetes. Equally, giving sugar to a Type 1 diabetic with low blood glucose levels can potentially stop them going into a coma or save their life. You may not be diabetic, but these two scenarios can serve as the catalyst for a mindset shift around sugar, and that's what's important. It's too easy to label high-sugar foods as 'bad' and yes, if you eat too much, you'll have energy issues, potential mood disorders and are nearly guaranteed to be above a healthy weight. That being said, if a small amount of sugar every day in the form of a chocolate bar is allowing you to adhere to your calorie-controlled nutritional plan, then I'd argue that it's quite a good food choice in this context. By the same token, if you are in a caloric deficit all week, eating mostly high-quality food from Monday to Saturday; and then you eat a full tub of ice-cream on a Sunday night to psychologically and metabolically keep yourself on track for the upcoming week, then that's quite a positive overall approach in my opinion.

If you are looking at this purely from a health standpoint, then the argument is different. I'm not going to link any of the tens of thousands of studies out there about how bad sugar is for you, as most of us know that too much sugar can lead to diabetes and obesity, or (as is less known) diminished virility, accelerated aging and potentially shortened life span. Instead of being another person telling you to cut back or eliminate all processed sugar, I'm just going to implore you to use some common sense. The danger really is in the dose: 10 chocolate bars every day will lead to problems, as will a tub of ice-cream every single night, rather than the considered doses mentioned above. Now I'll transition into a related topic that isn't as cut and dried: the story with fructose, aka fruit and its sugar content.

Fructose and fruit: the facts

Fructose is a monosaccharide component of sugar that naturally occurs in fruits. In that form, it is accompanied by cofactors that allow proper digestion and utilisation. I generally recommend fruit on any weight-loss plan. Of course you need to consider the calories (like every food) and the impact the sweetness levels can have on portion control: the sweet nature of fruit can make it easier to overeat, compared to say its nutrient-equivalent vegetable cousins, but generally it's a good option.

Some people have an aversion to fruit on a weight-loss plan and if you would feel more comfortable avoiding it, then do so. However, if you have a natural sweet tooth, then fruit can be a brilliant counterbalance to those sugar cravings. The sugars are all natural and are great on-the-go snacks. But if you think you would be more likely to succeed on a weight-loss programme by excluding fruit, then exclude it. If you enjoy fruit, have a sweet tooth or struggle with healthy snack ideas, then include it in your plan.

Which brings me on to something else that many people find confusing: industrial fructose. Examples are crystalline fructose or high-fructose syrup, which can be found in sweets, confectioneries and full-sugar drinks. Thankfully, if you're like me and living in Ireland, high-fructose corn syrup is banned, but if you live or are travelling in a country where it's available, be mindful of it. Another source of fructose (widely available in Ireland and the UK) is agave syrup, derived from the agave plant. Fructose products have a sweetness level that is higher or equivalent to that of sucrose; but agave syrup is much higher in fructose than plain sugar, so it has greater potential to cause adverse health effects, such as increased belly fat and fatty liver disease. Like everything, small doses and moderate intake are probably fine; but if you're living in the US and drinking soda every day or living in Ireland and drowning your pancakes in agave syrup, I'd probably look into alternative food choices.

Why is industrial fructose so bad? I'm glad you asked. It messes with your body's metabolism, as it bypasses the insulin response and devastates organs that are insulin dependent, such as the liver. The liver, whose sugar metabolism is insulin dependent, isn't programmed to utilise fructose, and therefore becomes extremely vulnerable to fructose accumulation. Desperate to prevent such accumulation and speed up fructose clearance, the liver converts it to lipids (fat), most of which are dumped into the blood circulation, with the remainder staying in the liver. It's like filling a bottle of water that's already half full. If you keep adding more water to it, it's going to overflow faster. In the same vein, too much overflow is essentially the problem with the fructose, fat and your liver.

The consequences of fructose accumulation include elevated blood lipids, fatty liver and can potentially increase your risk of obesity. It's not to say that you should completely avoid all industrial fructose, but if you've been mindlessly eating it (as its sweet taste can be addictive), thus leading you to overeat extra calories, it's worth nipping the problem in the bud and removing or greatly reducing your intake. As I said, whole fruits are perfectly fine, they have been an essential part of the human diet for centuries and are thus viable, tolerable and even a good food option for most people. Industrial fructose, not so much. A lot of people can get the two mixed up so hopefully this clears it up.

Salt: the facts

We've all been warned about the dangers of salt. Epidemiologists – the people who are on the scene to investigate disease outbreaks or other threats when they emerge – have highlighted the potential problem since the 1980s and, for the last 20 years, governments have been encouraging us to reduce our intakes through nationwide campaigns, food labelling and educational initiatives. The link between salt and blood pressure has been postulated for years and seems logical, as adding salt to water increases its pressure. In the 1990s, a series of observational studies showed that salt levels in the diet mirrored blood pressure, and when people with low salt intake and low blood pressure migrated to new locations with high intakes of salt, their risk of high blood pressure increased. Until I interviewed Tim Spector, the Professor of Genetic Epidemiology at King's College London, for my podcast and read his book, *Spoon-Fed: Why Almost Everything We Have Been Told About Food Is Wrong,*' I never really questioned that data.

His book explained about the growing body of evidence that some people respond much more strongly to salt than others, and are known as salt sensitive. The relatively new concept has caused some controversy as to whether salt sensitivity is a separate sub group or disease or part of the normal spectrum of how we respond to food, similar to dairy and lactose mentioned earlier. The reason I bring this up is to question the commonly held belief that 'salt is bad' – again, generic labelling of a food without any context. If you've just run a half marathon in the scorching sun, and you have sweated a large amount, ingesting or consuming some salt is likely going to be very beneficial in this scenario. If you have a history of blood pressure and are adding spoonfuls of salt to every meal, that is likely going to end badly. Context of the situation matters.

I remember the first time my family went abroad when I was nine or ten. I spent hours in the sun playing football with some Spanish and English friends that I met. Thankfully, I've always had quite sallow skin so I don't burn easily, but I do sweat quite a lot. I remember by day three, I had a pounding headache that just wouldn't go away. I was drinking water throughout the day and I wasn't sunburnt, but I couldn't get rid of the throb in my head. My parents weren't sure what was going on and were a little concerned that their otherwise healthy and active 10-year-old was complaining of a random headache that didn't seem to have any cause. My mother mentioned this to a couple by the poolside bar and they recommended I get a bag of crisps. Now, I'm not and never have been a huge crisp or chip lover. I always veered towards the sugary options like chocolate or ice-cream, especially on holiday; but lo and behold, within 20 minutes, I felt perfect again. Were crisps the magical cure for headaches? Well not exactly. Over 15 years later, when I was studying to become a sports nutritionist in London, I was completing a module about salt, sodium and electrolytes, most notably, the negative effects of dehydration or electrolyte imbalances for sporting performance. In this module, I came across the term 'acute hyponatremia', a condition characterised by low levels of sodium in the blood, and I recalled my time in Spain. Although it's impossible to say if I was at any real risk or danger, it did make me question for the first time the common belief that 'salt is bad'. As with so many things in this book, I'm not saying that salt is good or bad. What I am saying is that avoiding it completely, which I've seen several of my clients do (before working with me), without any good reason, is nonsensical. Some of them told me that they eliminated salt completely in the hopes that it would support their weight-loss journey. True, avoiding salt-laden foods could help you with your calorie deficit, but eliminating it completely without reason isn't a great idea.

As someone who sweats quite a lot when I work out, especially in hot weather, I always add a few pinches of pink Himalayan salt to my post-workout meal. If you are similar, then consider doing the same. Obviously if you have a history of high blood pressure and are concerned for your health, consult your doctor first. The message here is to question the common belief that 'salt is bad' without any context. When you understand that thinking that way about salt isn't very serving, it makes it easier to apply that same principle to everything you 'thought' you knew about diet, nutrition and food. When it comes to salt and all the advice you see in this book, or anywhere else, don't apply black and white thinking to a topic that is grey. I advise you include salt in your diet if you think your body needs it, i.e. you sweat a lot or live in a hot country, or you limit it if you have pre-existing issues. As with all the foods being examined in this section, remember:

1. Assess the context of your situation.
2. Question if it helps you with your end goal.
3. Apply whether to include it.

To listen to my podcast with Tim Spector, go to *www.briankeanefitness.com/the-keane-edge/bonuses*

MSG: the facts

There are two kinds of MSG: industrial and natural, apparently with opposite effects on the body. Industrial MSG is a flavour-enhancing salt, commonly added to food products such as bouillon or stock cubes, meat tenderisers, spice flavouring products, canned food, frozen foods, snack chips, sauces, instant soups and fast food.

My main issue with MSG is its highly addictive property and as you have probably gathered from the food list above, it's not generally added to any highly nutritious foods. MSG binds to opioid receptors in the brain that makes the food taste better and promotes overeating. If you've ever eaten Pringles or listened to their slogan 'Once you pop, you can't stop', this is probably one of the most common examples of the effects of MSG and addictiveness. If you've ever found yourself halfway through a full can of Pringles, wondering if you're ever going to feel full, then you've experienced this 'the more I eat, the hungrier I feel' phenomenon.

To avoid overeating due to the MSG content of certain pro-cessed foods, I advise you check the labels for their presence. It's normally listed under the following names.

- Hydrolysed yeast (in flavourings and spices)
- Protein hydrolysate (in sport nutrition products and infant formulas)
- Starch hydrolysate (sugar alcohol ingredient in low-carb products)
- Maltodextrin (in all kinds of processed products)
- Artificial flavouring (in diet, sport nutrition and baking products)

- Caseinate (in protein powders and bars, dairy products, ice-creams and baked goods)
- Whey protein hydrolysate (in poor-quality sport nutrition products)
- Aspartate (in supplements, meal replacement and nutrition bars)

Naturally occurring MSG

Unlike industrial MSG, natural MSG is a product of natural fermentation. In very small concentrations, it can have a hormetic effect (see chapter on stress for more on hormesis). Naturally occurring MSG, mentioned later in the supplement chapter when we discuss probiotics and pre-biotics for gut health, include: kimchi, sauerkraut, yoghurt, kefir and cocoa. All of which can potentially boost your defences and benefit your health, wellness and waistline in a calorie-controlled plan.

Simply put, industrial MSG should be avoided or at least minimised, while natural MSG has a whole host of potential benefits if you decide to include these foods in your plan.

Sugar alcohols and protein bars: the facts

Sugar alcohol is a common ingredient in low-carb or diet products and protein bars. Too much can cause bloating and in larger quantities, a laxative effect. The main issue with sugar alcohols is that they are extremely indigestible. I'll share a 'too much information (TMI)' story that expands on this. In 2014, I was preparing for the Miami Pro fitness model competition; for those unfamiliar with these competitions, think Arnold

Schwarzenegger bodybuilding show mixed with a Baywatch beach body competition and you have it. Anyways, nine weeks before the show, I had an increased craving for chocolate. This isn't uncommon during a competition prep, but on this occasion, it was particularly bad. My nutritional knowledge at the time clearly had a gap when it came to poly and sugar alcohols too. I went to the local supermarket and bought a chocolate-flavoured protein bar. Thinking I had made a 'healthy' food choice, I headed towards the exit. I wasn't yet at the automatic door when I found myself staring down the bottom of an empty protein bar wrapper, so I did what every logical person does at that point, I turned back and bought another bar. Then another, and another. Before I knew it, I had eaten six bars in total!

Now anyone who has eaten six normal chocolate bars in a row will know that you'll feel a little sick afterwards. Nothing too extreme, but definitely far from 100 per cent. This was another monster entirely. Within the hour, my stomach swelled up and I looked like I was six months pregnant! I also didn't have a bowel movement for three days! Three days! That was my first (and thankfully my last) experience when it came to over-consuming sugar alcohols. The bloating side effects of sugar alcohols aren't only unpleasant, they can lead to metabolic toxicity over time.[8] When it comes to fat loss, it gets worse, I'm afraid. A study published by the *Journal of Clinical Endocrinology & Metabolism*[9] revealed that sugar alcohol feeds certain gas-forming gut microbes known as methanogenic archaea, which cause obesity in animal and human models. These gut microbes produce methane gas, hence the bloating side effects. Now this isn't to scare you off them completely. Like everything, context and quantity matters – the occasional diet or protein bar is not going to leave you bloated, obese and toxic, and it's up to you whether you want to include them in your plan or not.

The only issue I have with protein bars, apart from the sugars alcohols, is they can sometimes be marketed as a 'healthy' food option. Healthy is a very subjective term. Healthy compared to what? Arsenic or a head of broccoli? Are most protein bars healthier than a deep-fried chocolate bar? Probably. Are they healthier than an apple or banana? Generally, no, and their nutritional choice comparison should be to that of a chocolate bar and not a piece of fruit. Some days, I'd prefer the sweeter sugar alcohol-filled salted caramel protein bar and other days, I'd prefer the normal sugar-filled treat of a milky chocolate bar. Just realise you're comparing protein bars to chocolate bars and the difference is very little in terms of nutritional value. My recommendation is to choose whatever you prefer and factor it into your nutritional plan.

Diet drinks: the facts

This topic has long been contentious for fitness professionals. Some argue that diet drinks are worse than their full-sugar alternative and the ghrelin-affecting, hunger-inducing effects of the sweeteners make you hungrier and increase your cravings more than if you just drank the original full-sugar version. Others preach them as a modern-day dietary life saver for individuals on a weight-loss plan because of the zero caloric value and the sweet taste's impact on nutritional adherence. I bet you'll never guess what I'm about to say? The truth lies somewhere in the middle. There are so many gut microbiome and individual variabilities to consider, that to conclusively say you should or shouldn't drink diet drinks is impossible at the minute. The answer is some people should completely avoid them and others will have no problem including them in moderation.

Let's talk about the negatives first. A study published in the journal *Nature* revealed that non-nutritive sweeteners, like the ones found in diet drinks, not only fail to provide the expected benefits of sugar replacement, they actually promote obesity and diabetes-related disorders more aggressively. Now I am hesitant to include any study that so blatantly falls on one side of the argument, as I never want to be accused of cherry-picking data to support a viewpoint; but this particular study was insightful for me and was the original one that shifted my mindset, so I'll go on. The researchers administered commercially available doses of saccharine (Sweet'N Low), sucralose (Splenda) and aspartame (Equal) in the drinking water of mice. The results showed that after 11 weeks, the artificial sweeteners-fed groups developed marked glucose intolerance, greater than that of the sugar-fed groups. According to the study, the obesity and diabetes-related side effects were caused by activation of sweet gut receptors that over-spike insulin and even more so by the disruption of gut bacteria. Translation, diet drinks can increase food cravings. The reason I have a soft spot for this study is that it eventually led me to the research[10] of how artificial sweeteners can wreak havoc on your gut microbiome. As someone with a history of gut issues and who spent years consuming diet drinks to save calories, this really opened up my eyes.

In 2015, I did a 180-degree turn on diet drinks. At the time, I was not a fan of them, full stop. I've since done a further 180-degree turn based on new evidence and currently think that diet drinks are perfectly fine (in moderation) for most people on a weight-loss journey. If, however, you have a history of stomach issues and gut problems or find that your cravings are significantly elevated when you consume diet drinks, I would cut back or possibly eliminate them completely. I'm afraid I can't put my hand on heart and say that every single person should avoid them. I also can't do the same to say they are perfectly healthy as those long-term studies haven't been done yet. What I can say is that if having a diet drink every day or a few times a week is helping you with your weight-loss goal, include it. If it's not or you have any of the issues mentioned above, then I would avoid it. Simple as that.

Saturated fat: the facts

Earlier in the book, we listed examples of monosaturated, poly-unsaturated and saturated fat. Of the three, saturated fat is the one that tends to get the most focus or publicity, partly because it's the fat that splits opinions on whether it's beneficial or unhealthy for your body and partly because it's largely misunderstood. Saturated fat, similar to salt mentioned earlier is another one of those 'let's just lump into the "bad" category without any context'.

We've already discussed the vital role fat plays in the body, and at the time of writing, there's a glaring lack of evidence against natural saturated fat, the kind found in food sources like red meat, egg yolks and real butter. An analysis in the *American Journal of Clinical Nutrition* evaluated more than 20 studies with a combined pool of nearly 350,000 subjects for proof of a connection between saturated fat and heart disease. The investigation found that there was 'no significant evidence for concluding that dietary saturated fat is associated with an increased risk of heart disease'.[11]

Over 20 years ago, my Irish household, convinced by government guidelines and possibly some television advertising, made the switch from eating butter to low-fat spread made with what appeared to be Italian olive oil. The television advertisements in the late nineties generally had pictures of Italian families, looking young, fit and healthy spreading margarine on their bread as they all dined in familial delight. But my grandfather was having none of that. He was a smart man and ahead of his time. A cattle farmer until the day he died, he had no intention of changing the diet habits of his father and his father's father before him because of some television advertisement; any time I went to visit his house, he had real butter in his fridge. I remember sneaking over to his house after school on several occasions just to make a sandwich with real butter. As a kid, I didn't care about the government guidelines or how happy an Italian family looked on TV, I just preferred the taste of real butter. As I got older and entered my teenage years, I become more 'health conscious' and inevitably made the switch to margarine. 'Well, they say it's healthier,' were the words I would say to myself. Oh, the famous 'they' who know everything.

Then like many things in this section of the book, something happened that made me question what 'they' had told me. I started to become more educated in how to read nutritional journals and interpret data from studies and a few things didn't add up. About six years ago, a few dissenting voices around the world began to question the wisdom of telling people to avoid butter. As you can imagine, there was a backlash, and what should have been a sensible scientific debate was inflamed by newspapers, articles and online debates accusing the authors of 'religious fundamentalism'. One of my early mentors used to warn me about giving out nutritional advice to those who aren't willing to hear it, regardless of how true or scientifically supported my argument was. She would regularly tell me that it's easier to change someone's view on religion than their views on nutrition. I can't speak to the former but as I started to consume these online debates in 2015/2016, I could definitely be convinced of the latter. As I mentioned earlier, I try not to cling too stubbornly to my nutritional beliefs. Even when interviewing individuals on podcasts who have extremely dogmatic nutritional beliefs, I try and approach it with Aristotle's philosophy, 'The sign of an educated mind is the ability to entertain a thought without accepting it', so when it comes to this particular topic, I think some people should limit their saturated fat intake and others should increase it. My goal here is to make you question what may have been a previously held belief and see if you need to discard it because it's no longer serving you.

When it comes to saturated fat, the first thing you need to do is not tar it all with the same brush. Egg yolks, butter and red meat, although high in saturated fat, cannot be nutritionally compared to pizza, biscuits and cakes, which are high in calories and low in nutrients. On the other hand, egg yolks, butter and red meat are much more nutrient-dense, making opportunity cost rear its ugly head again. The current recommendation is that foods containing saturated fat should be replaced with either starchy carbohydrates or unsaturated fats. This means, for example, that we should swap butter for low-fat spreads (the rebranded name for margarine). The desperate wish to have a simple message applicable to everyone – such as 'reduce all saturated fat' –

creates an obvious problem. This reductionist approach ignores complexity and quality of foods or dietary patterns, and it totally neglects context specific to the individual.

One of the more solid counter-arguments I get from clients is that low-fat spreads are lower in calories than their full-fat alternatives. Similarly, eating only egg whites saves on calories. I can't really talk here – In my earlier gym days, I would always remove the egg yolks when making scrambled or poached eggs, my thinking being that the egg white has all the protein, and the fat from the yolk is extra calories I don't need. Although logical, this was my nutritional ignorance at its finest. As important as calories are, the nutritional value of the food you eat matters a great deal. I hope at no point in this book do I come across as a 'calories in, calories out' coach. Yes, calories are important; they're the foundation pillar on to which your weight-loss pyramid will be built. But they're not the only thing that matter. If that was the case, I'd open the book with 'calculate your maintenance calories, get into a deficit and ignore everything else'. So when it comes to saturated fat in natural foods, my advice is not to avoid them. Obviously with a weight-loss goal, be mindful of their caloric value, but most well-rounded plans will include them in some capacity.

As for my personal choice, I realised a few years ago that my grandfather was right. When I graduated from university and moved into my own house in my early twenties, I threw away my pot of polyunsaturated vegetable spread with a tiny amount of low-grade olive oil, preservatives and yellow food colouring, and retuned to good old straightforward Kerrygold butter. The choice is yours, but at least now you have all the available information to make an educated decision based on your individual goals.

Trans fats: the facts

When it comes to trans fats, you need to start by asking if are you talking about health and wellness or fitness and weight loss. Based on the argument, my answer is going to be slightly different. The consumption of partially hydrogenated oils, which began in the early 1900s and increased during the 1940s, may have played a major role in the development of heart disease – long before we began blaming saturated fat. That much has become pretty clear over the past decade. Partial hydrogenation involves hardening oil, or any fat that softens at room temperature, into a never-melts, never-moves, tasteless solid to increase its shelf life. Nothing too crazy so far; a bit unnatural, I agree, but no more so than protein bars and diet drinks, and both of those are generally fine in moderation. So why the concern about trans fats?

Partially hydrogenating the liquid fats from soybean oil, corn oil and canola oil only adds to their long process of refinement. This makes them somewhat toxic to your body.[12] If this book was purely about health and wellness, then this would be an entire chapter in itself. When it comes to weight loss as a primary goal, the reason trans fats are so unsupportive towards your goals is the array of high-calorie and low-nutrient foods that they appear in – baked goods, cakes, cookies, pies, microwave popcorn, frozen pizza, refrigerated dough such as biscuits and rolls, fried foods, doughnuts and sticks of margarine. Not exactly a recipe for weight loss.

I've somewhat lightened my opinion on trans fats in recent years. In my first book, *The Fitness Mindset*, I was highly against them and although I still minimise them in my diet (especially fried foods and takeaways), I think the danger is again in the dose when it comes to a weight-loss goal. If 80 per cent of your food is nutritionally dense, then you probably have leeway with the other 20 per cent. Of course, if you're talking primarily about health and wellness, then it's a different conversation. In her book *Eat The Yolks,* author Liz Wolfe described the partial hydrogenation process as: 'the process of beating an already unhealthy oil into partially hydrogenated submission', or making a bad thing worse. So if your goal is health, wellness and longevity, I'd probably avoid them completely.

It's important to note that artificial trans fats, similar to MSG mentioned earlier, are not the same as the naturally occurring trans fat called conjugated linoleic acid (CLA), which is created in the digestive system of grazing animals such as grass-fed cattle. CLA concentrated in the fat tissue of these animals is widely known to support metabolism.[13] This is another reason why grass-fed beef can be a supportive food for fat loss, once you've considered its caloric value of course. It's also worth adding that CLA supplementation for a weight-loss goal has only been proven to reduce fat in rats,[14] so if you're a human being, the evidence is quite inconclusive at the minute. That's not to say it won't become clearer over time, but for now, I'd probably save your money and buy some caffeine or green tea extract instead. See page 152 for more on this.

Supplements

THE ROLE OF SUPPLEMENTS

Before we delve into what supplements will best support your weight-loss journey, it is important to approach supplements the right way. This leads me to the final gorilla in the room. There is no, and I repeat, *no* supplement that is a magic pill for weight loss. Your nutrition, your exercise regimen and your mindset all play a much more important role than any supplement ever could; but there are some that will support your journey going forward.

Everybody has individual supplement needs based on their nutrition. If you have recently been on a course of antibiotics, you probably need to consider a probiotic to re-establish the percentage of good bacteria in your gut. If you are following a vegan diet, as mentioned earlier, you are not going to be able to get vitamin B12 from plant sources alone; therefore, you will need a B12 supplement. If your diet is deficient in red meat, pumpkin seeds or other zinc-rich food sources, then it is worth considering adding a zinc supplement to your regimen. This is effectively what supplements are for. They 'supplement' what you are missing in your nutritional plan. However, the supplements I am going to recommend are specially designed to support a weight-loss journey. I have also chosen these supplements as they are scientifically backed and have been proven not to cause a 'rebound' or any major negative side effects when and if you stop taking them.

There are other more potent and powerful fat-burning supplements on the market than the ones I am about to mention. However, most of these are loaded with stimulants, to increase energy output that helps you burn more calories. Also, they generally include appetite-suppressing ingredients, so you eat less throughout the day. Not only do I dislike these supplements due to the negative rebound and side effects that appear when they either stop working or you discontinue use, but they are the complete antithesis to this book. Anything that sounds too good to be true or promises a quick fix should be avoided like the plague.

With all that taken care of, here are the three supplements I would consider adding to your arsenal for the next several weeks or longer as needed. Please note that you should always consult your doctor before starting any new supplement.

1. Caffeine

Caffeine is a staple ingredient in many popular fat-burning and pre-workout supplements. It primarily helps you to reduce body fat in two ways:

- **By boosting your metabolism.** Ingesting caffeine jumpstarts the process of lipolysis, which is when your body releases free fatty acids into the bloodstream to be used for energy. In other words, caffeine boosts your metabolism and can help you burn fat.

- **By giving you an energy boost.** One thing that everyone knows about coffee and caffeinated drinks or pills is that caffeine is a pretty strong stimulant. It increases alertness and wards off drowsiness temporarily, which means you can perform certain tasks more efficiently for longer on caffeine.

This applies for physical tasks as well as mental tasks. This means a little shot of caffeine can give you the energy you need to give 100 per cent during your workout. And giving 100 per cent in the gym means you will get the results you want more quickly.

Dosage

If you do not regularly ingest a lot of caffeine, a couple of hundred milligrams or a strong cup of black coffee will likely produce noticeable effects. You may want to start with 100mg to see how it goes and then up your intake to 200mg. You can then increase the dose by 50mg if you are still not experiencing any effects. Do be careful not to overdo it, as the side effects of a caffeine overdose can range from anxiety and insomnia to – in the most extreme cases – death.

Take 30 minutes before your workout to release free fatty acids to be burnt while you train, and to increase physical and mental alertness. However, be aware that caffeine has just over a five-hour half-life; so, if you take it too late at night, it can negatively affect your sleep. This means that if you consume 200mg of caffeine at 12 p.m., 100mg will still be in your system at 5 p.m.

2. Green tea extract

Green tea extract is probably my favourite fat-burning supplement. It has a low-to-moderate dose of caffeine, and it has another ace up its sleeve – polyphenols. These incredible polyphenols are supportive for any person trying to get lean.

In the scientific community, polyphenols are more commonly known as flavanols or catechins. The main catechins in green tea are epicatechin, epicatechin, 3-gallate, epigallocatechin and the one with the highest concentration, epigallocatechin-3-gallate, or EGCG. EGCG at a level of 45 per cent or more (the percentage is on the ingredient list of every green tea extract supplement) has the ability to do the following:

- Increase 24-hour energy expenditure, burning more calories throughout the day;
- Increase the body's key fat-burning hormone, norepinephrine, increasing the rate of fatty acid mobilisation;
- Prolong thermogenesis, increasing core temperature to burn more calories;
- Provide powerful antioxidants;
- Support a healthy immune system, stopping you from getting sick.

Dosage

For both men and women, taking between 500mg and 1,000mg of green tea extract (with 45 per cent or more ECGC) first thing in the morning or 30 minutes before training will support fatty acid mobilisation and increase metabolism for the rest of the day.

3. Acetyl L-carnitine

Acetyl L-carnitine plays an essential role in transporting fat into mitochondria – the furnace of the cell – where it can be burnt for fuel, which basically means it moves fat from the back of the queue to the front to be used as an energy source. Without adequate L-carnitine, most dietary fats cannot get into the mitochondria and be burnt for fuel. This is one reason why L-carnitine is considered a 'conditionally essential' nutrient – your body produces it, but if it does not produce enough, your fat loss can get seriously affected. Acetyl L-carnitine is slightly more expensive that L-carnitine tartrate, so if you're on a budget, consider the latter, as it works in a very similar way.

Supplementing with acetyl L-carnitine alongside caffeine and green tea extract can dramatically speed up your weight-loss goals without having too much of a negative effect on your central nervous system. If you think of your metabolism as a fire, caffeine and green tea extract can make the fire burn brighter, and L-carnitine pushes the fat into the fire to be burnt as fuel.

Dosage

For both men and women, taking 1–3g of acetyl L-carnitine first thing in the morning or 30 minutes before training can work very effectively.

VITAMIN D – THE VITAMIN THAT ACTS LIKE A HORMONE

Although regularly called a 'vitamin', vitamin D acts much more like a hormone on the body. We've evolved in the sun, and vitamin

D is a chemical workhorse that our biology came to count on. The body synthesises it after sun exposure, and it's activated by the liver and kidneys. That activated form acts like a hormone to regulate calcium metabolism. Some of vitamin D's many duties involve dampening the pro-inflammatory response and defending your cells from general wear and tear.

Although getting out into the sun for several hours a day is always the best option, it's just not feasible for some people based on their indoor job, lifestyle or the weather in the country in which they live. If supplementing, just remember: it's possible to have too much vitamin D in your blood. Vitamin D increases the absorption of calcium, and the major risk of vitamin D toxicity is hypercalcemia, or too much calcium in the blood. This can lead to problems such as kidney stones, along with other potential issues. On the other hand, it's impossible to get too much vitamin D from the sun – just remember to take proper sun precautions and not to burn.

While there is not a consensus on the ideal level of vitamin D, keeping blood levels in the range of 40 to 60ng/ml seems to be in the safe realm for most people. I have lived in Ireland for most of my life and I get my blood work done every winter to check my vitamin D levels. Then, based on the results, I supplement back in the amount I need to meet my daily requirements. This has worked wonders for my 'winter lows', something I suffered from when I was younger during the long, dark winter months. Your doctor can easily check your levels with a routine blood draw.

Dosage

Dosage should be 2,000 to 5,000 IU of vitamin D3 per day. This should be checked every six months by a doctor to ensure levels between 40 and 60 ng/ml.

RECOVERY SUPPLEMENTS

Although weight loss, fat reduction and your mindset in general have been the primary focus of this book, recovery should not be underestimated. If you are following the HIIT or gym workout samples from this book, or any other programme for that matter, the faster you repair from workouts, the better you will generally feel. One misunderstood element of recovery is its impact on your NEAT activity when combined with a resistance training programme. If you are following a weight or bodyweight workout programme, the chances are that you are going to be quite sore in between sessions if you are not prioritising your recovery. Being sore in between sessions normally leads to less movement throughout the day – your NEAT activity. If you have ever had a workout or joined a class only to find yourself struggling to walk the following morning, you know exactly what I am talking about here. If you are sore, you are less likely to stand at your desk, park further away from a shop to get extra steps in or just move in general.

Of course, 95 per cent of your recovery is down to your nutrition and sleep, but supplements are the final 5 per cent and can be the difference between feeling like you have been hit by a truck compared to feeling great after your workout session. When it comes to recovery, there is no need to reinvent the wheel.

Adequate protein intake is the foundation for any recovery plan. When it comes to this, here are the three options I recommend. Bear in mind that I personally think high-quality protein powder is all you need, but I'll also cover the other two for information.

1. Whey protein or alternative protein powder

The numerous benefits of whey protein include increase in muscular strength and size, decrease in body fat and a faster recovery time. Muscle protein synthesis is a scientific phrase thrown around a lot, which basically means that this synthesis enables muscle growth and is an important process for increasing muscle size and strength or building lean muscle tissue (toning up).

Resistance training alone can increase rates of protein synthesis. However, it also increases rates of protein breakdown. To build lean muscle tissue or to tone up, you need to tip the scale in favour of protein synthesis while trying to minimise the breakdown. Consuming whey protein post-workout can substantially increase muscle protein synthesis. Whey protein is a fast-digesting protein that enters the bloodstream rapidly. This allows it to get to your muscles faster and create a bigger spike in protein synthesis compared to food sources.

Dosage

The amount you use can vary depending on your body weight and protein requirements, but 25–50g per serving for men and 10–25g per serving for women 30 minutes after exercise is a good starting point for recovery. Alternatively, it can serve to increase protein intake throughout the day by adding it to recipes such as smoothies or protein pancakes. You do not really need to worry about the brand either. As long as your whey (or rice, hemp, soy, etc.) protein meets these three criteria, then you are good to go. The following are to help you choose the right protein powder for you.

- **A protein powder that digests well for you.** Some people have an issue with dairy, lactose or both. Others struggle to digest some plant protein sources so make sure that your protein powder is not causing you any stomach discomfort. If it is, it is probably a sign that you are not tolerating it well and should seek an alternative.

- **A protein powder that you enjoy the taste of.** There are so many great-tasting protein powders on the market, so experiment and find one that you enjoy the taste of.

- **A protein powder that fits into your budget.** Price does not necessarily equal quality when it comes to protein powder but low-price powders made with poor-quality ingredients can cause stomach discomfort in some. On the flip side, it should not break the bank either so find one that fits into your budget.

2. Branch Chain Amino Acids (BCAAs) and essential amino acids (EAAs)

The BCAAs are made up of three essential amino acids: leucine, isoleucine and valine. They are essential because the body is unable to produce them from other amino acids, so they must be ingested through food or supplements.

A large percentage of dietary amino acids are oxidised and wasted even before reaching the circulatory system. The exceptions to this pattern are BCAAs, with over 80 per cent of dietary content of leucine, valine and isoleucine reaching circulation.

EAAs include all three BCAAs plus seven more: L-arginine, L-histidine, L-lysine, L-methionine, L-phenylalanine, L-threonine and L-tryptophan. Whey protein is naturally high in BCAAs and contains all the EAAs, but for those who prefer to consume a capsule or who just dislike protein powders, try adding 3–5g depending on your bodyweight before, during or after your workouts to improve your recovery.

The studies on whether BCAAs or EAAs are more effective is massively split; so my advice would be to experiment with both and see which has the greatest impact on your recovery and then use that as feedback whether to continue or discontinue it. I rotate between both, but still favour a protein powder for its variety of use and cost effectiveness. Like everything in this book, it is about finding what works best for you.

Dosage

The dose varies depending on your bodyweight and training programme, but a good starting point is 3–5g pre- or post-workout.

DIGESTIVE ENZYMES AND PROBIOTICS

One of my mentors used to tell me that, 'It's not about what you eat, it's about what you absorb,' and when it comes to using digestive enzymes or probiotics to support that theory, it's largely true. As we discussed earlier, your food choices matter a great deal; but if you are making good-quality food choice but still struggle with random bloating, digestive issues or just a general feeling of fullness after meals, then these might be the supplements that support you with those issues.

'Probiotic' is the term used to describe microbes that are good for us. It's worth adding that, although most common probiotics are a type of bacteria, some are also yeast. According to Dr Megan Rossi, author of the #1 Sunday Times bestseller *Eat Yourself Healthy*, to 'fulfil the probiotic definition' there are three main criteria:

- The microbes must be alive.
- They must be present in large numbers.
- They must have evidence of a health benefit.

As someone who battled with irritable bowel syndrome and gut issues for most of my early years, I've been using probiotics to support my gut health for nearly a decade. However, there are so many variables to consider when choosing the correct one for you. Different probiotics do different things and therefore have different effects on different people. It's like medication – you wouldn't take a painkiller to improve your cholesterol. Probiotics are generally the same.

When it comes to choosing a probiotic, I advise either getting an expert gut doctor to support you or alternatively you can test it yourself. When you introduce a probiotic, it typically takes about four weeks or longer to see any noticeable effects; but if you find that your mood is enhanced, your energy levels are improving and your digestion is greatly improved, there's a good chance that the probiotic you have chosen is working well for you. Most probiotics can be taken with or without food but always check the label first. When selecting a brand, I recommend choosing one that has a reputation for creating high-quality products. Dissimilar to the supplements mentioned earlier: caffeine, green tea extract or acetyl-carnitine, where dosage is more important than brand; when it comes to probiotic selection, you generally get what you pay for. From my experience, most low-priced probiotics tend to be low quality and moderate or higher-priced ones tend to have higher colony-forming units (CFU/day), so check out reviews and talk to experts to find the best one for you.

Don't confuse prebiotics and probiotics!

A prebiotic, not to be mistaken for a probiotic, is essentially food that feeds specific beneficial microbes. The main prebiotics include inulin, fructo-oligosaccharides (FOS) and galacto-oligosaccharides (GOS). These are found in over 35,000 plant species from apricots, dates, dried figs or mango to asparagus, almonds, rye and dandelion or fennel tea. The reason I want to differentiate between the two is that I am *not* recommending you take a prebiotic supplement. Taking advantage of the naturally occurring prebiotics in food is absolutely the best way to feed your gut microbiome. If your nutritional plan includes lots of fruits and vegetables alongside healthy fats and complex carbs such as nuts and grains, you should be adequately covered in the prebiotic department. Of course, individual cases may need individualised plans, so if you have a goal that's deeper or more intricate than general weight or fat loss, I recommend you consider working with a professional who can design a plan specific to your needs.

To listen to my podcast with Dr Megan Rossi, go to *www.briankeanefitness.com/the-keane-edge/bonuses*

Digestive enzymes

When digestive issues like bloating, gas, nausea, constipation or diarrhoea are a regular event after eating, it can put a serious dent in your quality of life. While it's comforting to know you're not alone – a lot of people suffer with similar issues – when those pesky and sometimes downright painful symptoms strike, you'd like to experience some actual comfort too. Although I'm a fan of digestive enzymes, one of my primary concerns is, although they can work very effectively at supporting the issues listed above, they can equally be used to paper over any cracks in your overall nutritional plan. For example, if you have an issue digesting milk due to a lactose intolerance, you can take a lactase enzyme to minimise the discomfort felt when eating or drinking those foods. Alternatively, you can seek out different food choices such as coconut or almond milk. I can argue strongly for both scenarios; but when it comes to sustainability, creating new dietary habits that don't require a supplement for absorption tends to win out in the long run.

What are digestive enzymes and how do these supplements work?

The body secretes a variety of enzymes to break down the foods that we eat—some are secreted starting in the mouth; others start further down in the digestive tract. The most important enzyme categories are the proteases (which break down proteins), lipases (fats) and amylases (starches and sugars). Normally the functioning glands in the mouth, stomach, small intestine, gall bladder and pancreas are professionals at producing the enzymes we need to digest our food and absorb the subsequent nutrients properly – but when these glands are either non-functioning or have been damaged, digestive enzyme supplements are intended to help pick up the slack.

Who might – or might not – benefit from taking digestive enzyme supplements?

People with conditions like irritable bowel syndrome (IBS), inflammatory bowel disease or low stomach acid might find digestive enzyme supplements helpful. Equally, individuals on the other end of the spectrum such as professional athletes, ultra-marathon runners or anybody who works out for multiple hours a day generally need support with their digestion too.

But if you don't have a definite enzyme deficiency (you can find out for certain by having your poop tested), or your symptoms are more of a nuisance than severe, it might be easier on your wallet to simply remove any foods from your diet that are causing digestive distress in the first place. For most people, removing sugars, grains, liquid dairy or industrial seed oils from the diet can dramatically improve the digestive issues many might try to treat with a supplement.

Choosing a digestive enzyme supplement

The over-the-counter digestive enzyme supplements on the market are modelled around the three primary categories of digestive enzymes that are created naturally within the body (protein-, fat- and carb-specific). Two of the more well-known examples are lactase, mentioned above (for digesting lactose found in dairy products), and alpha-galactosidase supplements (for sugars found in cruciferous veggies and legumes). There's also a number of supplements that contain a combination of digestive enzymes and claim to alleviate multiple gut issues at once. Similar to choosing a probiotic, high-quality reputable brands are a good starting point. After that, it's about experimenting and testing it for two or three weeks to see if it removes or reduces the issue you need addressed.

Things you should know but shouldn't focus on

People ask me questions all the time, but at the end of the day, the answers to many of them just don't matter all that much, and you'll see why shortly. However, all these things have some basis and warrant a conversation – unlike stuff like skinny or diet teas, sauna suits or most infomercial quick-fix fat-loss gadgets or machines.

Below are the ones that you have probably found yourself asking about at some time or another. If not and you are a complete beginner, these are the ones that tend to come up quite early on during a fitness journey. Although useful, they fall into the 'majoring in minor things' bracket, and play such a small role in your overall progress that spending time educating yourself around them is only going to yield marginal gains. But let's go anyway.

1. BODY TYPES/SOMATOTYPES

Identification of different body types, or somatotypes, is usually based on an assessment of your stature, muscle and fat mass. The approach was defined by an American psychologist, William Herbert Sheldon, in the 1940s. Sheldon coined the terms we still use today: ectomorph, endomorph and mesomorph. An ectomorph will have a tall, light build, small joints and lean muscle. A typical endomorph will have a shorter, squarer build, and can easily gain fat. The traits of the mesomorph are a typically athletic shape that responds quickly to training, with visible differences soon apparent.

My point isn't to argue against the body type classifications – they are very useful starting points when trying to identify your genetic starting point or what way your body is inclined to respond based on the nutrition or training programme you follow. However, like everything in this section, although useful information to have, I also wouldn't worry too much about it. Making high-quality food choices, looking after your mindset and finding a workout regimen that works for you is always going to be the best approach.

Ectomorph – is this you?

Naturally long and lean, you might find it hard to gain weight, and increasing your exercise can mean you lose fat and end up skinnier than you want to be. You might be familiar with the term 'hard gainer', which is gym slang for someone who is naturally skinny and struggles to add size. This is your typical ectomorph. To build size and strength, try to include compound exercises which use more than one joint or muscle group. Eating high-quality carbohydrates such as brown rice, sweet potato or oats alongside good-quality fats: olive oil, nut butters, etc. can help to ensure you don't lose weight as you work out more. Consistency with food is absolutely crucial with an ectomorph, albeit for the opposite reason to an endomorph. A typical ectomorph could lose months of gym progress in a week (if they get sick, for example) and can become very disheartened. This will only be temporary though, and the weight should climb up again once you go back to your regular eating plan.

Endomorph – is this you?

You might already be blessed with an 'hourglass' or 'V' shape, and you should also find it easier to gain muscle when you integrate resistance training into your exercise plan. Circuit training or HIIT should work well for you. It's also worth including some cardio work, be it jogging, swimming, cycling or focusing on your step count in your fitness regimen so that you maintain the right level of body fat too. Nutrition is also key for an endomorph. If you are genetically inclined to gain weight easily, it's worth being a bit more mindful of your food choices and overall calorie intake. This is slightly less important for a mesomorph or ectomorph, but should be pretty high on your priority list.

Mesomorph – is this you?

If you are lucky enough to be predisposed to a naturally athletic build, your body will typically respond well to weight training and you will see the changes fast. Try to include some multijoint workouts that include lots of compound lifts and potentially some sports like tennis or swimming which work your whole body. Similar to endomorphs, keep an eye on your nutrition, because although you will gain muscle pretty easily, you are generally inclined to gain fat as well if your calorie intake is too high.

2. FITNESS WATCHES/TRACKERS

This one is a little trickier for me to break down, for two reasons mainly. One, I love my fitness watches and devices; but as a fitness professional who keeps up to date with the research and anecdotally experiments with them, I am keenly aware of their limitations. The second reason is down to a basic understanding of Moore's Law and the rapid speed of technological change. The next few sentences, unlike the other 99.9 per cent of the book, are likely going to be out of date soon. Considering that, I shall attempt to give you the advantages and disadvantages of fitness watches and trackers, alongside their limitations, while also predicting where they may evolve or be addressed over the coming years.

Advantages

- **Accountability.** A fitness tracker encourages you to exercise every day, whether it's walking, jogging or working out. It can make you more committed to getting your steps in or completing your workout sessions. My favourite thing about my fitness watch is using the step count to hit my 10,000-a-day target. You can also use a phone app for this, but a watch is considerably easier and you're unlikely to forget to turn it on as it normally starts when you strap it to your wrist in the morning.

- **Motivation.** A fitness tracker gives a visual of your progress and accomplishments each day, and seeing this progress is good motivation to improve more and more as the days pass. I hesitate to put any predictions forward in this book as the majority of its content and information is trial-tested and scientifically backed or at the very least, heavily anecdotal, in the examples of mindset or client case studies. That being said, I think gamification of fitness will be one of the biggest trends we see over the next decade. The accomplishments, games and visual representation of your progress after hitting a step count target, for example, is only going to evolve over the coming years.

- **Healthy eating.** I've already stressed the importance of a healthy diet in conjunction with exercise. Using an application to track your food and water intake can help you maintain a healthy lifestyle. MyFitnessPal is currently my favourite app to track food, but it's largely individual preference, as most calorie trackers are pretty much the same.

- **Goal setting.** With a fitness tracker, you can set goals for yourself to accomplish each day – for example, 10,000 steps a day. I also find tracking your runs or cycles on various apps can also be very useful in helping you hit a specific time or personal best. Strava is my current favourite for tracking my running and cycling.

- **Heart rate monitoring.** Most fitness trackers have the ability to monitor your heart rate by measuring your pulse, allowing you to reach your target heart rate with each workout. They can also detect changes that may occur to your heart rate. The general best practice to calculate your maximum heart rate is to subtract your age from about 220. During moderate physical activities, your target heart rate is about 50 to 70 per cent of the maximum heart rate; with vigorous workouts it should be about 70 to 85 per cent of the maximum heart rate. It's worth noting that the accuracy of different heart rate monitors can vary greatly, and you generally get what you pay for here. A free app will generally be less accurate than a fitness watch, which will generally be less accurate than a €300 monitor you wear while you exercise. Once you are aware of this, they can be a useful tool to give you feedback on the difficulty level of certain exercises regimens or workouts. This is especially true if you are a beginner and not fully in tune with your body yet.

Disadvantages

- **Expense.** Fitness trackers can be expensive to buy. I generally recommend that you don't buy something based on price, buy it based on value: 'buy cheap, buy twice'. You are better off saving and buying a €200 watch that you really like, and use every day, versus a €50 watch that you never use. I'm not a financial advisor, but a good rule of thumb for any purchasing decisions you make is to buy things based on the value you get and not the price you pay.
- **Battery life.** Most trackers have limited battery life. When charging your device, you will not be able to keep track of your steps or workouts. I feel this will be addressed in the coming years, but at the time of writing, it's a disadvantage.

- **Accuracy.** Some trackers do not provide 100 per cent accurate metrics/information – some of the information shown on the device is just an estimate. Try not to fully rely on these devices. Calories burnt is currently one of the metrics that I highly recommend you avoid. At the time of writing, they are only slightly better than randomly throwing darts at a board and picking a number. This will doubtless improve in the future, but be mindful of it now.

- **A need to unplug.** There are some fitness trackers that include WiFi and Bluetooth. This allows you to receive incoming calls, text messages or emails without looking at your phone. For some people, this falls into the advantage list, as it's a great way to stay connected without always being close to your phone. For me, however, it's a disadvantage. As someone who regularly does digital detoxes to improve my overall happiness and wellbeing, fitness trackers (and your phone) can disrupt this, with the feeling of always being 'on'.

- **Sleep tracking.** At the time of writing, this is currently a disadvantage, as most trackers are wildly inaccurate when it comes to tracking your sleep. However, with the current research that is ongoing, I'm confident that fitness trackers will soon have the ability to track your sleep patterns, how deep or light you sleep, how long you slept, and each time you woke up, in a very accurate way. Recognising your sleep patterns can allow you to have a good night's sleep and improve your mood the next day. Watch this space.

3. EATING AND TRAINING AROUND MENSTRUATION

This isn't to underplay the role of premenstrual syndrome (PMS) and lower the focus on the hormonal changes that happen during your cycle every month. In fact, for the women I work with who get monthly cravings and really struggle the week before or week of their period, I'm a big fan of 'calorie cycling'. This is a very similar approach to carb cycling mentioned earlier in the book when breaking through weight-loss plateau, but instead of cycling carbohydrates on different days, you cycle your calorie intake on different weeks.

For example, let's say your cravings for chocolate surge every month before your period. You know it, I know it, the whole world knows it. It's set in stone and it's like clockwork for you and your body. Seven days pre-period, you would give your left arm for chocolate. In this context, increasing your calorie intake with a chocolate bar or two, or with whatever food you're craving, the seven days leading up to your period can be a very effective approach. Let's use this very simple example to go deeper with this.

Your maintenance calories are 2,000kcal per day. Anything below that is a calorie deficit – we covered this in Part One. Now let's say you want to eat 1,800kcal per day: that's a 200kcal-per-day deficit. You could do this by eating 1,800kcal every day for week 1, 2, 3 and 4 for the month, or you could cycle those calories with 1,600kcal each day for one week, 1,800kcal for two weeks and 2,000kcal for one week. Both ways maintain a deficit, but one allows for more leniency on the week you struggle with cravings.

Sample month

- Week 1: 1,600kcal
- Week 2: 1,800kcal
- Week 3: 1,800kcal
- Week 4: 2,000kcal (cravings week)

Of course, I'm using these arbitrary numbers to illustrate a point. You might want to have a few chocolate bars that week and bump your calories to 2,300kcal in week 4 and then drop them to 1,300kcal in week 1, or you can mix and match. It really doesn't matter as long as you maintain your caloric deficit over the month. This can be a very effective strategy if you know your cravings are going to be worse on some days compared to others.

I should also note that hormonal cravings due to your time of the month is very different from generic cravings that regularly occur. This is normally down to a nutrition, lifestyle or sleep issue, and needs to be solved at the root; so don't confuse the two.

4. TRAINING SPLITS

I'm not saying that training splits – the way you break up your workouts through the week – are unimportant. In fact, following a training programme specific to your goal is very important. However, when it comes to training splits, the actual consistency of your workouts is more important than the routine you follow. That being said, below is a breakdown of the more popular body composition splits.

Push/pull/legs split

This is a personal favourite of mine, and is actually the training split from my first book, *The Fitness Mindset*. The reason I like it so much is down to its time-saving warm-up element and its significant rest between training a body part a second time that week. To explain, your 'push' workout constitutes all your muscles that require that movement pattern – chest, shoulders, triceps, calves, etc. Pull workouts constitute back, rear delts and biceps. Legs then generally make up glutes, hamstrings and quadriceps. Because you are training similar biomechanically designed muscle groups together, you can decrease your workout time by saving several minutes on warm-ups.

For example, if you are doing a bent-over row for your back, you are simultaneously warming up your rear delts and biceps in the process. This translates to less time warming up each muscle group, and can get you in and out of the gym (or home gym) faster. The other major positive of this split is that it allows for quite a long rest period between training a body part a second time, thus potentially optimising recovery, from a training standpoint anyways. If you are doing five days in the gym, for example, your split might look like this:

- Monday: Push
- Tuesday: Pull
- Wednesday: Legs
- Thursday: Push
- Friday: Pull
- Saturday: Rest
- Sunday: Rest

Or alternatively, if legs or lower body are of a higher focus, it might look like this.

- Monday: Legs
- Tuesday: Push
- Wednesday: Pull
- Thursday: Legs
- Friday: Push
- Saturday: Rest
- Sunday: Rest

Either way, you are getting a 48–72-hour rest before you train a body part a second time, and this can allow for maximum training efficiency due to the enhanced recovery between sessions. This has been my favourite training split for nearly 10 years, and although I experiment with the others mentioned, I always come back to it as my foundation pillar for training.

Upper/lower body split

This is pretty self-explanatory. One day you train your upper body, the next day you train your lower body, and you repeat this continuously. It works quite well if you're training for fewer days. In an upper/lower split you can have a highly intense workout on lower body one day, repeat it with upper body the next day; then rest and recover. Then you repeat this a second time in the week for a total of four workouts. A typical upper/lower split would look like this:

- Monday: Upper
- Tuesday: Lower
- Wednesday: Rest
- Thursday: Upper
- Friday: Lower
- Saturday: Rest
- Sunday: Rest

I've never been a huge fan of this split for several reasons.

1. The warm-up time is considerably longer than a push, pull and legs split, as you generally have to warm up each of the major muscle groups (chest, back, shoulders, etc.) separately to reduce your risk of injury.

2. The intensity of the workout tends to reduce as your session progresses. The reason push/pull/legs can be so effective is because you generally start with the bigger muscle group (chest on push day, back on pull day, quads on leg day, etc.) and then gradually move to smaller body parts as you fatigue. You can do this with upper/lower too; it just tends to be less effective in my opinion.

3. I find that the workout can be extremely demanding if you do it more than four times per week, so if you're similar to me and enjoy working out five days a week, this may not be the workout split for you.

That being said, if you enjoy it, then I recommend you make that the foundation of your training plan. Also, similar to all the splits mentioned, you might train at the weekends. I'm just using the sample weekly layout for simplicity.

Full body split

Another one that is pretty self-explanatory: you train your full body in each workout. This programme is very effective if you focus on your compound lifts (squat, deadlift, military press, rows, bench press or glute bridge, etc.) and can only train a few times a week. I generally recommend this to those who can't commit to more than three sessions per week. This way, you can utilise a full rest day in between each workout to counteract the intensity of training your entire body on a single day. A typical upper full body split would look like this:

- Monday: Full body workout
- Tuesday: Rest
- Wednesday: Full body workout
- Thursday: Rest
- Friday: Full body workout
- Saturday: Rest
- Sunday: Rest

This is generally my 'go-to' workout split on especially hectic weeks where I'm working to deadlines or have life or family commitments that mean I can't fit in any more than three workouts that week. It's a useful approach if time is short or you struggle to prioritise more workouts. Combining it with 10,000 steps a day and a calorie deficit makes it a fantastic split for a weight-loss goal.

Body-part split

Also known as a 'bro split', although equally applicable to women, this is where you choose a body part and train it in a single day.

A typical male split might look like this:

- Monday: Chest
- Tuesday: Back
- Wednesday: Shoulders
- Thursday: Arms and abs
- Friday: Legs
- Saturday: Rest
- Sunday: Rest

A typical female split might look like this:

- Monday: Glutes
- Tuesday: Quads and hamstrings
- Wednesday: Shoulders
- Thursday: Back
- Friday: Arms, chest, abs
- Saturday: Rest
- Sunday: Rest

The obvious benefit to this split is that you can increase the volume that you approach any individual muscle group and really focus on the composition for that body part. For me, I always found that I fatigued too quickly on this type of training programme and could never get the most out of any individual workout unless I combined it with something like a CrossFit metcon (metabolic conditioning) or a bodyweight circuit at the end. For example, if I was training my back, my first couple of exercises like rows or pull ups would be great, but then my back would be so tired that I'd be incredibly weak for the second half of the session.

Of course, there are so many variations of these workout routines and so many more; but these tend to be the ones I see most often. Like everything in this book, it's not 'one size fits all'; it's very much about finding what works best for you and doubling down on it. Experiment with the ones I've mentioned above and see what you like the most or what fits best into your schedule. The best workout split is going to be the one that you can stick to. That also tends to be the one you enjoy the most. It's also worth reemphasising that if weight loss is your primary goal, any activity that helps you burn calories is going to play a more important role to your progress than the actual split you follow; so do what you enjoy – just make sure you do it consistently.

5. FASTED CARDIO

I can sum this up easily: does fasted cardio suit your lifestyle? If yes, do it fasted. If not, do it post-workout or at another time of the day. It has been hypothesised that performing aerobic exercise after an overnight fast accelerates the loss of body fat, but the research[15] just doesn't support that claim.

When it comes to fasted cardio and your ability to lose fat faster by incorporating it, I've changed my opinion on this in recent years. When I was competing in fitness model shows where my primary goal was fat reduction and muscle preservation, I was pretty firm on my opinion that fat loss occurred more quicky if fasted cardio was implemented. Granted, I had seen several studies that showed it made no difference as to what time of the day you did your cardio; but anecdotally and from personal experience, my mind was set.

Unfortunately, as I regularly see with personal trainers

nowadays, that also meant that my belief system at the time was generally projected onto my clients. If one of my clients wanted quicker fat loss, I added in fasted cardio to their programme. Generally, it worked; but not because it was fasted or first thing in the morning. It worked because their output had increased, i.e. they were burning more calories with the increased cardio, so fasted cardio become a self-fulfilling prophecy loop. It wasn't until 2014, when one of my girls flat-out refused to do fasted cardio, that I opened my mind to alternative viewpoints. She didn't oppose fasted cardio for any scientific or moral reason, she just refused to get up 40 minutes earlier to do cardio before her workout. She liked her sleep and was damned if any personal trainer was going to mess with that. I remember the conversation like it happened yesterday.

> **Laura:** Brian, I am *not* getting up 40 minutes earlier to do cardio!
>
> **Me:** Okay, what do you propose then, will we reduce your calorie intake?
>
> **Laura:** Well, can I not just do the cardio after my workout or when I got home from the office?
>
> **Me:** Well, I suppose you could, but you won't be fasted so it might not work as well.
>
> **Laura:** Okay, I'll do that instead.
>
> **Me:** We'll test it next week, but just so you know, it might not work because you really need to be in a fasted state to maximise fat burning.

I face-palm my forehead due to my incredible scientific ignorance in this particular area every time I think of this reply. You can probably guess what happened next. We tested her body fat levels a week later. It was down. A week later, it reduced again, and that pattern repeated itself for six straight weeks. I remember thinking, 'How is this happening? Does she not have to be in a fasted state to tap into fat stores more efficiently?' Alas, no. As we've already discussed, cardio burns calories. Burning calories can support a calorie deficit. The timing really doesn't matter.

But are there benefits to fasted cardio versus doing it after a workout or at another time of the day? Of course. One is that you get yourself moving first thing in the morning, and that's always a good habit to get into. Two, it's quite time-efficient and is less likely to get forgotten. If you get up 20 to 40 minutes earlier to go for a walk or jump on a cross trainer, it's at the start of your day, so you're less likely to skip it because you're tired or a work/family commitment has come up. Which brings me back to my original question. Does fasted cardio suit your lifestyle? If fat loss is your primary goal and cardio is a component of that, does doing it first thing every morning before you've eaten anything serve that purpose? Or are you like Laura and won't get up earlier in the morning for anything less than love, money or gold? In that case, do it at another time of the day. A calorie deficit and your overall nutrition is the foundation pillar for your fat loss pyramid. Cardio is a few layers up, important, just not as important as your overall nutrition. Which ultimately means that you should go for your walk, set the treadmill to incline or jump on the cross trainer whenever suits you best. It really doesn't matter too much as long as you get it done. Consistency with it is significantly more important than the timing of it.

6. INTERMITTENT FASTING

Mentioning fasting as a way to lose fat generally gets one of two responses. As I write, intermittent fasting – where you periodically eat for a given window of time during the day (say eight to ten hours) and then you don't eat for the other 16 to 14 hours – is quite popular in weight-loss circles, and for good reason. If you're trying to get into a calorie deficit and you reduce your eating window to eight to ten hours, you're likely to consume fewer calories. If you consume fewer calories, your chance of going into a caloric deficit goes up. If you're in a caloric deficit, you lose fat. That's effectively intermittent fasting and fat loss 101 for how or why it works.

Of course, there will be some other secondary benefits too: improved insulin sensitivity means you utilise your carbohydrates more efficiently; potentially better digestion through the eating break that comes with fasting can make you more metabolically flexible, but why it works so well for fat loss is just common sense. If you give yourself less time to eat, you're likely to eat less. It's similar to going to a golf course for an hour versus for a whole day. If you're trying to hit a hole in one, I'd put my money on the person who's doing it for 24 hours versus the single hour. Neither person is necessarily guaranteed to hit a hole in one; similarly, intermittent fasting is no guarantee for fat loss, especially if you are consuming too many calories during your eating window, but your chances of success potentially go up.

A response I generally get when I mention intermittent fasting is a pessimistic eye roll. When I say 'fasting', people hear 'starvation'. 'So you're going to starve me?' No. That's not it at all. Fasting is completely different from starvation in one crucial way:

control. Starvation is the involuntary abstention from eating. We dispelled the myth of your body going into 'starvation mode' earlier, and a more accurate case of starvation would be the World War II concentration camp victims or the prisoners in the Gulags in Stalinist Russia. Starving people have no idea when and where their next meal will come from. This happens in times of war and famine, when food is scarce. Fasting, on the other hand, is the voluntary abstention from eating, in this example, to support a caloric deficit. Food is readily available, but you choose not to eat it. Some people experience hunger when they go into a caloric deficit, that's normal; although this isn't a hard-and-fast rule, as your food choices play a major contributing factor as to how you feel in this situation. However, when people start intermittent fasting first, in my experience, nine out of ten people tend to experience increased hunger initially. Similar to fasting, hunger and starvation are also not to be confused. Assuming you are well fed generally, hunger won't kill you, and normally passes over like a wave in time. Starvation can kill you, and it's important to understand the difference if you are considering using intermittent fasting as a weight-loss tool.

You may begin a fast at any time of your choosing, and you may end a fast at will, too. You can start or stop a fast for any reason, or for no reason at all. Fasting for weight loss has no standard duration – since it is merely the absence of eating, any time you are not eating, you are technically fasting. For example, you may fast between dinner and breakfast the following day, a period of 12 or even 14 hours. In that sense, fasting is already a part of your everyday life. Consider the term 'breakfast'. The word refers to the meal that 'breaks your fast' – which is done every single day. If intermittent fasting is something you want to try, but its application worries you, it's worth rewiring the way you even see the word. The word itself implicitly acknowledges that fasting is performed daily, even if only for a short duration. It is not something strange, but a part of everyday life.

Do I recommend intermittent fasting?

Well, that depends. Like everything in this book, it's about finding what works best for you. Intermittent fating is just another tool that you could potentially use – don't overcomplicate it. Skip breakfast or dinner one day a week and see how you feel. If you find yourself overeating at the next available meal – the main downside to intermittent fasting where fat loss is concerned – try going with a shorter gap between meals next time. A popular weight-loss strategy is to fast for 16 hours every day and eat for eight hours. For example, you might have breakfast at 10 a.m., lunch at 1 p.m., a snack at 3.30 p.m., dinner at 5:30 p.m. then fast until 10 a.m. the following day again. As long as you're maintaining your deficit, this is a very efficient way to lose body fat. It's especially useful if you find that you're not really hungry when you wake up anyway and regularly find yourself skipping breakfast and heading straight out the door in the mornings.

But remember you can't just eat whatever you want in your eating window and expect to lose fat. As obvious and silly as it sounds, you can't eat a 3,000kcal surplus every day with chocolate and pizza and expect to lose fat, even if you're following intermittent fasting protocol. If you hear somebody telling you otherwise, please ask them to show you a single study that supports that claim. None currently exists, and I doubt any ever will.

As always, if it works for you and supports your end goal, keep it. If not, discard it and try something else.

7. THE KETO DIET

The ketogenesis diet, popularly called the 'keto diet', is one that puts the body into a ketogenic stage. But ketogenesis is actually a function of human physiology in which the body uses fat for fuelling muscular contraction, organ function and the general activities of daily living. We shift into a ketogenetic state in the absence of glucose. This can happen with fasting; the process is typically well underway when going without food for 18 hours or more, or when eating a diet high in dietary fat, low to zero carbohydrate and low protein. While a 'keto diet' focuses on what nutritional choices you can make to maintain a ketogenic state even while continuously eating, this diet isn't necessary to get the benefit of ketogenesis. As mentioned in the fasting section above, you simply need to be void of digestible calories to start using your own body fat as fuel. Technically, you could potentially eat a pure carbohydrate diet but fast for 18-plus hours and still potentially become ketogenic. I don't recommend this, but I think it illustrates the point that to enter ketosis, you have two ways of doing it – through diet or through fasting.

Do I recommend a keto diet?

Generally not. Other than for those with epilepsy, as the research[16] for the ketogenic diet is strong in that instance, I'm not a fan of this protocol for those looking to lose fat. This is partly due to its incredible restriction of food choices, but also because you need to really educate yourself on the difference between nutritional ketosis, fasting ketosis and physically testing your individual ketone levels alongside regular experimentation of macro splits and food choices to optimise your ketogenic state. In terms of difficulty, if counting your calories is like the game of checkers or drafts, following a keto diet isn't just like chess; it's closer to the 3D wizard chess that Harry Potter plays in *Harry Potter and the Philosopher's Stone*. There are so many moving parts to consider, and if your primary goal is fat loss, there are lots of alternative and more straightforward ways to achieve that goal. Also, due to its severe food restriction – no cake, bread or any foods you might enjoy – and its difficulty to adhere to in social settings – restaurants, drinks with family or friends, etc. – it's really hard for me to recommend it to anyone.

Another major issue I have with it is the misinformation surrounding the ketogenetic diet that leads some people into believing that they can eat all of the dietary fat they want – generally truckloads of butter – and still lose fat. As with eating whatever you like if you're intermittently fasting, this obviously isn't true, which some people unfortunately find out the hard way. Of course, if you want to experiment with the ketogenic diet, consider reading resources such as the book *Keto Clarity*, or following reputable ketogenic researchers like Dominic D'Agostino online.

Personally, I like regular intervals of going into ketosis myself if I'm training for an ultra-endurance event. But even as someone who considers themselves quite disciplined when it comes to nutrition, the thought of giving up all my favourite foods, never touching alcohol again or being the sap sitting there with a lump of butter at Christmas dinner just doesn't appeal to me. If you're struggling to lose weight or reduce your body fat and have any behavioural or relationship issues around food, I generally recommend you stay well clear of following one of the most restrictive and difficult-to-adhere-to diets of all time.

8. SLIMMING CLUBS

Slimming clubs are diet clubs where groups of people come together, digitally or in person, to help keep one another accountable. Most clubs have a 'leader' who guides the meetings, and its focal point is normally a weekly weigh-in on a weighing scale. If your weight is down that week, you get celebrated, if your weight is the same, or worse, has increased, you bow your head in shame and vow to do better next week. I will break down this negative association with the weighing scale that's reinforced by peer pressure in a moment. Spoiler alert though. This is the primary reason I don't recommend these clubs – especially if you already have a bad relationship with food. Having a poor food relationship and then signing up to a diet club is like digging a hole, trying to get out, but digging deeper in order to get yourself out – your poor relationship with food just gets worse and worse.

Outside of the negative mentioned above, most diet clubs generally give you a set of guidelines that aren't really based on any nutritional merit: a point system, a syns count or some other arbitrary metric. You might think that as a nutritionist, I'd scoff at this, and I kind of do; but not as much as you might think. I can see that the mass appeal of clubs like this is their simplicity. They are incredibly easy to follow. You don't need a bachelor's degree to apply the basic principles. For example, you get 30 points every day. A chocolate bar is 3 points. Cool, now you have 27 points left. A subway sandwich is 11 points. Great, you have 16 points left for the day. Pretty straightforward. But you also have 'zero-point' foods. Oh, don't get me started on zero-point foods. In one popular slimming club, boneless skinless chicken breast and all types of fish are pointless. So are eggs and kidney beans. Meaning you can eat as much as you want. It doesn't take a rocket scientist to understand how nonsensical this is. *All* food has calories, from chocolate bars to chicken breasts. Their macro and nutritional profile will be different, the chocolate bar will have more sugar and the chicken breast will have a higher protein value, but they both have calories.

You can see why this system is easy to follow and truthfully, it works for some people. Want to know why (although you may have already guessed it)? If you're 25 kilos overweight and your 30 points is enough to put you into a calorie deficit, you will lose weight. Also, if you're at the very beginning of a weight-loss journey and have gone from never making a conscious food choice in your life to now looking at food labels, chances are, you're going to become a more mindful eater. This can potentially lead you to eating less.

For me, it's not the lack of nutritional education that I find concerning. Not everyone geeks out on food like I do, and some just want a simple, easy-to-follow way to lose weight. I'm like that with my car. I don't care how my mechanic fixes it or what the underlying issue with the engine was, I just want little old Betsy to get me from A to B. My main unease with diet clubs is their disconcerting attempt to make people feel bad about their lack of progress, especially in a metric as variable as weight. Everything from carbohydrate intake, stomach contents (needing to poop), sodium levels, hydration and hormones (time of the month) can all make weight fluctuate day to day and even hour to hour. You may have strictly kept to your points tally all week, not overindulged on free foods and were in a calorie deficit for the seven days. If you measured your body fat levels, it would have likely decreased that week. But let's say hypothetically that you ate some cereal for breakfast (carbohydrates) and your lunchtime pasta had a little too much salt. You drank loads of water because of that damn salty lunch, and it's the week before your period (if you're female). You go to weigh in at the diet club at 6 p.m. and wham, you're up 1 kilo. You might then think, 'WTF just happened, I was so good all week!' and in most cases go home deflated, unmotivated and wonder why you even bother. This might even lead to a massive food blowout because you start to think, 'What's the point?'

Unfortunately, I've heard way too many variations of this exact story with clients I've worked with over the years; and that's what disturbs me about these clubs. The lack of nutritional education, although I don't agree with, I get it. Some people see food like I see my car, so I get that. What I can't get on board with is the lack of education on basic human physiology combined with the primary focus on one unit of measurement (weight and weighing scale in this case) to indicate progress. That's absolutely ludicrous. That's like judging the quality of the house by its floor and not looking at the whole thing – 'Ah yes, those are lovely floors you got there madam', not looking up to see that there's no frigging roof on the house!

Nutrition and weight loss need to be looked at as a whole. When you isolate things, like what happens when you only track weight for progress, you miss the whole picture. Slimming clubs are just houses with the roof missing. Better than living on the street, but give me a house with four walls and a roof every day of the week. Similarly, a diet club might be better than nothing, but give me a solid nutritional plan that's in alignment with your specific goals every day of the week too. Next time you are tempted to join a slimming club with its points systems and weekly weigh-ins, ask yourself, would you move into a house with no roof? If the answer is no, then you should probably avoid the slimming club, too.

9. VEGAN DIETS

Of all the diets or nutritional protocols above, this is probably the most difficult to break down from a nutritional standpoint, as it's a whole book in itself. Although I will attempt to discuss the pros and cons of following a vegan or plant-based diet, I should add that there are several great books out there on the topic, from *The China Study* by T. Colin Campbell and Thomas M. Campbell II to *The Plant-Based Power Plan* by T.J. Waterfall. Not to mention some fantastic vegan cookbooks, including *Vegan Cooking for Everyone* by The Happy Pear. I should probably clear up two things first. If you're vegan or plant-based for ethical reasons, then I have nothing more to add. That's your lifestyle choice and just as with someone's religion or spiritual beliefs, I'm not going to tell you what you should or shouldn't believe. That's your decision and I fully respect it.

The second thing is that 'vegan' and 'plant-based' are not the same thing. The only similarity is that both abstain completely from all meat, fish, eggs and dairy products; but those two diets can look very different. A vegan diet can be an incredibly low-nutrient plan with poor-quality food choices to make it up. You can eat dairy-free vegan ice-cream that's loaded with sugar. You can eat highly processed meat substitutes that are loaded with artificial colourings and flavourings. You can eat vegan cookies that are full of trans fats. Vegan doesn't equal healthy. It doesn't even equal low calorie most of the time.

Plant-based vegan nutrition is something else entirely. This plan is generally something that I do recommend to people on weight-loss journeys; although my professional opinion skews more towards a balanced approach of plants mixed with high-quality meats, fish, eggs and dairy (if you can tolerate it, see the dairy section earlier in the book for more on this). If you're sticking to wholefoods, with lots of nuts, seeds, fruits and vegetables, you are going to feel pretty damn good. Also, if you're tracking calories, you'll be shocked to see how much food quantity you can eat on a plant-based plan and still be in a deficit. The reason? Most vegetables are pretty low in calories. The same for most wholegrain carb sources like quinoa, oats or rice. It's not all upside though I'm afraid.

If you're planning to go fully plant-based, you need to know the key nutrients for vegans. Some people may require supp-lementation or using fortified foods to meet their nutritional requirements. This is certainly the case for vitamin B12. For vegans, considering your vitamin B12 intake is probably the most important message you need to take from this section. Vitamin B12 isn't produced by plants, but by microorganisms. In the case of meat, these microorganisms live in the stomach of the animals, and produce B12, which is absorbed into the bloodstream and accumulates in the animals' tissues. So for vegans, and most vegetarians, it's the one vitamin which absolutely must be taken either in supplement form or by eating foods that are fortified with vitamin B12. It plays a variety of important roles, ranging from DNA synthesis, red blood cell formation and the formation of myelin – the protective sheath that surrounds nerve fibres. Clinical signs of B12 deficiency can include fatigue and weakness due to a low number of healthy red blood cells, as well as tingling, numbness, memory loss and confusion owing to nerve cell damage. The real fear with B12 deficiency is if it's left unchecked over time, some of the neurological damage is irreversible.

Another thing to consider is that B12 is a water-soluble vitamin that can be stored in the liver for quite some time. So for people first adopting a vegan diet without suitable supplementation or fortification, B12 stores can slowly decline without showing any symptoms for many months or even years. This can lead to a false sense of security, believing that you don't lack B12, meanwhile deficiency can slowly creep up on you. The dosage recommendation varies from person to person, but it's generally thought that vegans should take a daily supplement providing at least 10ug or a weekly supplement providing at least 200ug. This is because the less frequently you obtain B12, the more you need to take, as it's absorbed better in small amounts. B12 is by and large the most important vitamin to consider for vegans; but if you want more details on what other vitamins you should look out for, I highly recommend reading *The Plant-Based Power Plan*, mentioned earlier.

My final point on a vegan diet is that it's not necessarily good for fat loss. We talked about dairy and gluten earlier in the book;

but a vegan diet and fat loss is very similar. Going vegan doesn't equal fat loss. In some cases, it actually equals fat gain because of the extremely processed nature and high caloric value of some of the vegan alternative foods. It depends what you replace your food with. If you remove eggs and replace them with Chinese vegan noodles, you now have a higher-calorie, lower-protein and poorer-nutrient food swap. Or for an extreme example, let's say you swap your grilled steak for a vegan cookie – you're going to have a problem. Remember just because a cookie is made without eggs and dairy does not make it automatically healthier or lower calorie – some vegan cookies can pack an incredibly high number of calories and sugar. However, similar to everything in this book, this isn't an anti-cookie message – quite the contrary! I'm all about balance and eating the cookie; but I'm just creating awareness here.

Do I recommend a vegan diet?

As you probably know by now, I'm a big proponent of including plenty fruits and vegetables, especially green/leafy ones, in your plan. The nutrient density in these foods is so high that it's difficult not to recommended them. But eliminating meat, fish, dairy and eggs entirely can cause its own problems. As long as you're aware of this and you're using the right food combinations, ensuring you're still meeting your protein requirements and staying in a caloric deficit, the only real question then is: do you want to go vegan?

If you want to experiment with it, you can try it one day a week, then increase it to two days a week until you potentially get to seven. Again, it's very much down to whatever is the best fit for you. If you think your life quality and waistline will be greatly enhanced by following a more plant-based lifestyle, then do it. If you think you're going to struggle by removing meat, fish, eggs and dairy from your plan, or the thought of that makes you feel uneasy, then I'd probably avoid it.

To listen to my podcast with The Happy Pear or T.J. Waterfall, go to *www.briankeanefitness.com/the-keane-edge/ bonuses*

Training

NEAT, HOME HIITS AND THE GYM

Although 80 per cent of your progress in a weight-loss journey will come down to your nutrition, I'd be remiss not to mention training. The primary goal of this section is to make you realise that when I say training or 'working out', I'm not talking about four or five one-hour gym sessions every week. That works great for some, but there are other ways in which you can derive the benefits of exercise.

First, there are non-exercise activity thermogenesis (NEAT) activities, which include walking, standing more or even things such as gardening, cleaning the house, going to the shops or having sex. Another way to think about it is *exercise that doesn't feel like exercise*. Then there are bodyweight HIIT workouts. These are a bit more structured than NEAT, but work great for fat loss and don't require a large commitment of time to receive the maximum benefits. Finally, there's the gym, which most of you are familiar with. I will touch on the pros and cons of all three, but it's about finding what works best for you, what you enjoy the most and what fits into your lifestyle and schedule.

Strategy 1: NEAT

Non-exercise activity thermogenesis (NEAT) is the energy expended for everything we do that is not sleeping, eating or sports-like exercise. It ranges from the energy expended walking to work, typing, performing yard work, undertaking agricultural tasks and fidgeting.[17]

Your metabolism is always working to burn energy. During periods of higher activity such as working out, your body will burn more calories than when you are at rest. However, even when you are at rest, your body is always expending energy. How you burn energy or expend calories comes down to your total daily energy expenditure (TDEE), which we discussed in Part One of the book. Your NEAT activity can serve as a great low-hanging fruit when it comes to lowering body fat. You can hit your weight loss target by just monitoring your calorie intake and focusing on your NEAT activity. No gym, no HIIT sessions – just some conscious effort to make small and seemingly insignificant changes to your lifestyle. As with the compound effect, it really adds up over time. Here are five tips that will increase your NEAT, to help you reach your weight-loss goal:

1. **Standing can make a difference.** A growing body of evidence shows that sitting still for too long can be hazardous to your health.[18] Simply standing is one form of NEAT that can help increase your daily caloric expenditure. I bought a standing desk for my office over a year ago; now I do all my writing

and work tasks standing throughout the day. If you work a sedentary job or in an office, see if there is a possibility to make this one small change.

2. **Daily steps add up.** The recommended number of steps you should take a day is 10,000. Although the origin of this dates back to 1964 and a promotional campaign for the Tokyo Olympics, there's a lot of research to suggest that this is a good target number to strive for each day. The reason I like it is because it's an achievable goal for daily physical activity for most people. Fitness watches or phone apps are a great way to track it too. Even if you don't make it to the 10,000-step target, adding extra steps to your day is an important component of NEAT that can burn calories while adding health-promoting activity to your life.

3. **Walking or cycling for transport is beneficial.** Have you ever been stuck in traffic during your commute and thought, 'There has got to be a better way'? By choosing to walk or ride a bicycle for your daily commute, you can burn significant amounts of energy during an activity in which most people spend their time sitting. If you take a bus or train as part of your commute, getting off a stop or two early provides a great opportunity for some extra walking. One of my early life fitness friends used to tell me that 'Driving to work makes you fat and burns through your money. Cycling to work makes you save money and burns through your fat.' Although there are obviously some limitations to this based on how far away you live from your workplace, it could be a very useful way to burn extra calories throughout the day.

4. **House cleaning and gardening help.** Doing additional tasks around the house or putting a little extra effort into your daily chores can be a great opportunity to increase daily NEAT. I'm a fan of habit-stacking this with my favourite podcast or an audiobook. I'll be a shameless self-promoter here and recommend *The Brian Keane Podcast* if your goal is weight loss, or if you have an interest in health, fitness or mindset in general.

5. **Play with your kids (or your family or friends' kids).** Assuming you or a family member has children, and you can carve out even a few minutes from your day to play catch, kick a ball or walk down to your neighbourhood park, you'll be spending precious time with your family while racking up NEAT. Personally, one of my rest days every week is an 'active rest day' with my daughter, so we're normally spending an hour or two swimming, playing football or just running around playing tag. It's a great calorie-burner, and in my opinion running after a six-year-old is harder than any leg workout!

NEAT pros

- You don't have to make any huge sacrifices to increase your NEAT.
- It can easily slot into your normal daily routine with some alterations.

NEAT cons

- The results aren't as noticeable as the other options listed below.

- It can be tricky to hit your step target on wet days, but I recommend kitting yourself out with a good waterproof jacket and doing it anyway. When it comes to hitting a fitness goal there's no such thing as bad weather, just bad clothing.

Strategy 2: HIIT

HIIT workouts generally combine short bursts of intense exercise with periods of rest or lower-intensity exercise. They can be done with weights, fitness equipment or your own body weight, which is my preferred method. Here's a sample HIIT workout that takes less than 20 minutes and will get you sweating and your heart pumping.

1. Air squat
2. Burpee
3. Mountain climber
4. Plank
5. High knees
6. Jumping jacks
7. Bum touches
8. Reverse crunch

Complete one minute of each, rest for three minutes, repeat twice.

HIIT pros

- You can do it at home in as little as 20 minutes a day.
- You can use your bodyweight as resistance, so you don't need to spend money on equipment.

HIIT cons

- It's harder to hit secondary goals (increase strength, build muscle, etc.).
- If you have a family or kids at home, it can be tricky to prioritise the time. In this instance, I recommend getting up half an hour earlier and doing it first thing in the morning before you start your day.

Strategy 3: Gym

This is probably the most well-known of the three strategies. You might have said to yourself, 'Oh I need to lose weight, I'd better join a gym', and for some people, that can work great, but it's not the only way. If you struggle to prioritise the time for the gym or have anxiety about working out around others, I recommend starting with either strategy one or two above, and then progressing to the gym whenever you feel ready.

When using weights, find one that you can lift for 10 repetitions. If you can do 11, 12 or 13 repetitions, the weight is too light, and you need to increase it. If you fail at 6, 7 or 8 repetitions, the weight is too heavy, and you need to reduce it.

Here's a basic sample gym workout that focuses on all your major muscle groups:

1. Barbell squat
2. Barbell deadlift
3. Military press
4. Dumbbell row
5. Dumbbell shoulder press
6. Bodyweight push-ups (from floor or full)

Complete 3 sets of 10 repetitions; rest for 90 seconds.

Gym pros

- It can be focused 'me time'; you go the gym, put on your favourite music playlist, and work out for 40–50 minutes, then you go home.
- There are lots of different weights and machines, so you won't get bored.

Gym cons

- You may have gym anxiety (the fear or worry that everybody is watching you when you are working out), and you may not feel confident about how to do certain exercises.
- It might not be the most time-efficient method, based on traffic, distractions from talking to other people and so on.

To download workout videos for HIIT or gym strategies for FREE, go to *www.briankeanefitness.com/the-keane-edge/bonuses*

WHAT'S THE BEST KIND OF TRAINING?

As I mentioned above, there are numerous different training systems and finding what works best for you is the key. However, when it comes to building a lean and toned physique, there are definitely a few things to consider.

Cardio or weight training for fat loss?

True, cardio is a very effective tool for fat loss because cardio can burn more calories than resistance training alone, i.e. you are more likely to burn more calories doing an hour of running vs an hour of resistance training. So that means you should do loads of cardio to lose fat faster, right? Well, not exactly.

In reality, cardio and resistance training both work for fat loss, just in different ways. Cardio can help you burn more calories during your actual workout session, which may support a calorie-deficit plan faster. Resistance training, on the other hand, can elevate your metabolic rate, so you burn more calories while you rest, or what I like to call the king of magazine clickbait (albeit true) – 'burn fat while you watch TV'.

Burn fat while you watch TV

Here's how weight training allows you to burn calories while you watch your favourite TV show. When you weight train or work with resistance in general, using body weight, dumbbells, bands or barbells etc., you tear muscle fibres. These fibres need repairing after every workout, for which they use calories from food and amino acids from protein. Instead of those calories adding inches to your waistline, training effectively gives them another job to do – repair from the workout. In order for your muscles to repair, your metabolism has to increase, lending itself to burning more calories while you rest. Resistance and HIIT are great systems for 'getting a better bang for your buck' because you do less to get more. Depending on the programme you are following, these torn muscle fibres could be repairing for up to 72 hours *after* the workout, and the food you eat can be going towards repair and not into fat storage.

That is not to say that cardio does not have a place, it certainly does. If you enjoy running, you should run. If you enjoy high-intensity workouts, then HIIT sessions are the way to go. When it comes to overall fat loss and training, the question is not 'What's the best cardio'; it's 'What do you enjoy the most and what can you stick to?'

If your goals change and your focus becomes more about body composition and toning up, then a resistance programme is going to support that more; but when it comes to fat loss, think consistency versus intensity. What cardiovascular activity do you enjoy the most? Make that the bedrock of your plan and be consistent with it. This might be anything from running, cycling, swimming and power walking to playing tennis, gardening and housework. Obviously, if you want to step it up a level and build a lean, toned and athletic physique, you should follow a resistance programme with some element of cardio – HIIT, step count or low-intensity cardio. Your training, similar to your nutrition, should be in alignment with your goals. Random training and random eating = random results, so get specific based on your goal.

Part Four
Sleep and Stress

Why sleep is important

Do you think you got enough sleep this past week? Can you recall the last time you woke up without an alarm clock feeling refreshed, not needing a cup of coffee to get going? If the answer to either of these questions is 'no', you are not alone. Two-thirds of adults throughout all developed nations fail to obtain the eight hours of sleep a night recommended by both the World Health Organization and the National Sleep Foundation. That probably doesn't surprise you. Most people, a younger version of myself included, have the default thinking that sleep is just something you have to do. You don't really need to prioritise it, it just kind of happens. It's funny, because if you just 'kind of' eat whatever you want, you just 'kind of' get fat. So why would random sleep patterns be any different?

Well, partly because we don't see the negative effects of poor sleep hygiene straight away. Yes, you have probably experienced a poor night's sleep and felt really tired the next day, but you probably didn't give too much thought to what happens over the long term. In this regard, it's exactly the same as weight loss or weight gain. You don't eat a 1,000kcal Big Mac and instantly gain 10 kilos. If you did, you probably wouldn't eat it. Smoking is similar: if you got cancer after a single cigarette, no one would smoke. Sleep is exactly the same – we generally don't see the negative effects of poor sleep quality until far into the future, at which point it's almost too difficult to come back from. As I said, you're probably not surprised that two-thirds of adults get less than the recommended amount of sleep, but you may be surprised by the consequences. Routinely sleeping less than six or seven hours a night demolishes your immune system, more than doubling your risk of cancer.[19]

When it comes to weight loss, inadequate sleep – even moderate reductions for one week – disrupts blood sugar levels so profoundly that you would be classified as pre-diabetic. Have you ever noticed your desire to eat more when you're tired? This is no coincidence. As you'll see later, too little sleep swells concentrations of a hormone that makes you feel hungry while suppressing a companion hormone that otherwise signals food satisfaction. Despite being full, you still want to eat more. It's a proven recipe for weight gain in sleep-deficient populations. Worse, should you attempt to diet or go into a caloric deficit but don't get enough sleep while doing so, it is futile, since most of the weight you lose will come from lean body mass, not fat. The less lean body mass or lean muscle tissue you have, the slower your metabolic rate and a decreased amount of calories burnt throughout the day. It's like the Red Queen in *Alice in Wonderland*: you have to run twice as fast just to stay in the same place. If you go into a calorie deficit but don't address your sleep issues, you'll have to diet twice as hard just to maintain your current weight. Not exactly a recipe for success.

I try to sleep eight to nine hours every single night. When I hit this target, my workouts are better, my heart rate is healthy, my nerves are sharp, my creativity or memory peak and I'm not walking around all day craving caffeine. That may seem like a lot of sleep to you, but as you've already seen, sleep is pretty darn important. If someone says they need fewer than seven hours, or less than the average person, 99 per cent of the time they are lying to you or to themselves, or both. As someone who has been a notoriously poor sleeper most of my life, I find it very easy to see how poor sleep quality can not only affect your waistline, but also your overall life quality in general. Poor sleep takes its toll on everything – from your energy levels in your workouts to your willpower and ability to make better food choices throughout the day.

See if this situation is in any way familiar. You wake up to your alarm on your phone and reach over to turn it off. While you're there, you check the notifications beamed in overnight from social media, the emails and texts from work and friends. Your mouth is dry, your brain feels like it's still somewhat asleep, there's light leaking in through the curtain while the TV, laptop or device light is on standby at the foot of the bed, staring unblinking at you, reminding you what you were watching right before you feel asleep last night. This was my morning routine for the better part of my twenties.

Having a basic understanding on how sleep works is essential to addressing the problem. True, I could jump straight into a topic like sleep supplementation and hope the quick-fix band aid addresses the issue; but just like painting a dead tree green and then saying it's alive, getting to the root issue is going to serve you much better. With that in mind, let's start with the problem of poor sleep.

THE PROBLEM OF POOR SLEEP

A lot of us waste time falling asleep and spend hours in a light sleep state that doesn't have the same body- and brain-boosting benefits of deep REM (rapid eye movement) sleep. In the past I would spend an hour trying to fall asleep because my brain wouldn't stop rehashing the day's events; this was especially true in my twenties, when I would replay all the conversations I had that day right before bed. Now don't get me wrong, this kind of self-evaluation can be a very positive thing: it tells you exactly where your life needs to improve and gives you direct feedback on what you have to work on. If you felt deflated after a particular conversation with a negative work colleague, you might make note to stay clear of them the following day. If you messed up on a work deadline because you were procrastinating on social media and are now doubly stressed because you need to fix it in the morning, you might think twice about randomly scrolling through your feed tomorrow.

This self-analysis is important and I'm a big fan of it generally, but while you're trying to wind down and fall asleep is not the time to think about it. If you're of the personality type that overthinks everything and replays the day's mistakes over and over in your head, my advice is to designate a time specifically for this and journal your thoughts. Even if you never look at it again, there's a mental cathartic release we can get from writing down things that we need to work on, and then leaving it or coming back to it in the future. I guarantee that if something is playing over and over in your head, writing it down will make you feel a lot better and reduce your overthinking or anxiety before bed. But if that doesn't work, and you're lucky enough to have a trusted and loving inner circle, you could instead try share those spiralling thoughts with a friend, partner or family member.

During my mid-twenties I actually started to feel like sleep was a waste of time. I tried different supplements, going to bed earlier, going to bed later, but I would still wake up groggy every morning and never really felt recovered. I'm not a sleep doctor, but I have spent years trying to figure out why I wasn't able to sleep better, and I've since been fortunate enough to have fixed the exact same problems with hundreds of clients that I've worked with over the years. There's really only one secret you need to know about sleep. The secret? It's not about sleep quantity; it's about sleep quality! Before I get into how to improve your overall sleep quality, it's important to first understand how you're evolved to sleep, and how things like blue light from your phone screen can stop you falling asleep from a physiological standpoint.

HOW WE'RE EVOLVED TO SLEEP

Let's start by going off the grid for a week or two. Let's get back to nature for real. Picture yourself leaving all your possessions behind – your digital watch, laptops and phones – and head out to an uninhabited part of the world where we'll live off the land, just as our ancestors did. We'll hunt, fish and sleep under the stars.

So out here in this part of the world, we set up a camp. When the sun eventually goes down, and the temperature drops with it, we build a fire and catch up about what happened during the day. Eventually after an hour of eating and chatting, the conversation gradually starts to subside and one by one, we turn over, curl up under our blankets or sleeping bags and drift into sleep.

At some point in the morning, depending on the time of year and the part of the world, the sun is going to start approaching the horizon, and when it does, the temperature starts to rise. You'll hear the birds starting to sing even before then. Even if it's really cold, the temperature will rise by a couple of degrees, and everything will get lighter. Whether or not we're all wrapped up in our sleeping bags, the natural light gets in and we wake up. The first thing we're likely to want to do is relieve ourselves and empty our bladders; after that we'll start thinking about food and what to have for breakfast, and before long, it'll be time for our morning bowel movement. Nothing rushed or hurried, all in its own time. This is how we're evolved to fall asleep and wake up – but to be honest, I've only experienced this exact scenario once. It was in 2018, when I completed the Marathon Des Sables in the Sahara Desert. With the exception of hunting for food, this was exactly how my routine was for eight straight days and nights.

It was the first time I had experienced a complete absence of electronics and artificial light and every night without fail, I fell asleep around 8 p.m. and woke up every morning with the sun at 5 a.m. Generally I don't need that many hours of sleep, but running a marathon a day in 40-to-50-degree heat made me more tired than normal, so I tended to need an extra hour or two each night to recover. That wasn't what got me thinking, though. I've been training for 20 years, and my sleep requirements always increase when my training volume goes up. The thing that struck me most was how good I felt every morning. Even though I was running a marathon a day for six days straight, because I was falling asleep when the sun went down and waking up when it came up, I actually slept better in the desert than I had at any stage in my life! It was an experience that got me very interested in understanding more about our natural circadian rhythm. I had mentally prepared myself for eight nights of terrible sleep, but the opposite happened: I ended up sleeping right through the night and waking with the sun feeling fully refreshed – or as refreshed as you can be after running a marathon the previous day.

Ever since, one of the first things I do with clients who are chronically poor sleepers is to ask them if they're aware of the circadian rhythm. Most have heard of it, but aren't sure what it means, and there's a good chance that if you're a poor sleeper, you may not understand it fully either. I didn't at first anyways.

A circadian rhythm is a 24-hour internal cycle managed by our body clocks. This natural clock of ours, deep within the brain, evolved over millions of years to work in harmony with the earth's rotation, and regulates our internal systems such as sleeping and eating patterns, hormone production, mood and digestion. Your internal body clock is set by external cues, daylight being the main factor. It's vital to understand that this circadian rhythm is hardwired in your DNA: trying to change your circadian rhythm is like telling a fish it needs to get out of the water and learn to fly, or a lion that it has to turn vegan. The best physical example you may have experienced because of your circadian rhythm is when you travel across different time zones and feel 'jet lagged'. When you go from the southern hemisphere to the northern hemisphere, for example, your body gets mixed up between night and day – that's why you're so tired during the day and so energised at night-time. Your body does reset back to normal and your internal body clock will self-adjust in the new country once it gets a few days of the day/light cycles in, but this phenomenon shows you how hardwired it really is.

The reason that I was able to sleep very early and so well in the Sahara was because, once the sun has gone down, a hormone known as melatonin starts to be produced. Melatonin is the hormone that regulates our sleep. It's produced in your pineal gland and responds to light. Once it's been dark long enough, we produce melatonin naturally and we're ready to sleep. This intuitive need to sleep starts building as soon as we wake up and becomes greater the longer we stay awake. That's why you're generally fresher in the morning than at lunchtime or the evening, as you haven't been awake as long. However, our circadian rhythm is able to override this at times, and that's the reason that we sometimes experience a 'night-time second wind'. Anyone who's ever worked a night shift or pulled an all-nighter for an exam can attest to this: even though you're exhausted after a full night of work, your body and brain still struggle to fall asleep during the day, as you're fighting your body's circadian urge to be up with the sun. Here are a couple of sleep hacks that night workers can use but, truthfully, they're for anyone who struggles with sleep in general. I use all of these nearly every night to ensure I get better sleep quality.

Sleep hacks for night workers

1. Get blackout blinds that completely block out all natural sunlight in your bedroom. The key is trying to recreate the

darkness of night-time in your room: if the sun is beaming through your window, you're going to struggle to fall asleep and to stay asleep. For a double dose of darkness, get blackout curtains as well. As a general rule one or the other will suffice, but I use both to ensure my bedroom is as dark as a bat cave.

2. Cut the screen time an hour before sleep – this is good advice regardless of what time you go to sleep. I also use 'blue light-blocking glasses' if I want to watch a film or some TV before bed. I'll cover more about blue light in a moment, but for now, cutting back on melatonin-blocking blue light can help you fall asleep more easily after having worked a night shift.

3. Fake a night-time routine. As a night-shift worker, it can be difficult to have one of these, as you're coming home when everybody else is getting up or still asleep. Routines are very powerful in subconsciously switching off from the day's events (or night's, in this case). Try and go to bed at the same time every day and keep the routine similar. For example, if you get home at 7 a.m. – eat, have a shower, watch an hour of TV, brush your teeth, go to your blacked-out room and sleep from 10 a.m. to 6 p.m. This is just an example, so adjust for your lifestyle and preferences.

The problem with blue light

Although there are other factors, light is the most important time setter for our body clocks, and there are very few things better than the daylight in the morning to help get you ready to get up and go. In the Sahara, sleeping under the sky, I got my fix as soon as I woke, but in the real world, it's very easy to spend our time indoors –at home, on the train or in our place of work and, in Ireland especially, overcast days are normally supported by the artificial lights at home or in the office. My advice is to get your curtains open as soon as you wake up, or use a daylight alarm clock that mimics daylight and wakes you by light instead of by alarm; I use this religiously in the winter and it's great for anyone who is affected by seasonal affective disorder (SAD), whereby your mood is negatively affected in the winter months from a lack of sunlight.

We are particularly sensitive to a wavelength known as blue light. This is the light that is emitted from electronic devices such as laptops, computers and smartphones. It's not that blue light is bad for you; daylight from sun is full of blue light and during the day, blue light helps keep you alert and awake. It naturally sets your body clock, suppresses melatonin production and keeps you focused throughout the day. But can you see how all those positive traits during the day quickly become negative if you're planning to sleep in the next few hours? Sleep expert Chris Idzikowski uses the great term 'junk sleep', which is where, even though you may be getting the traditional eight hours of sleep, the electronic gadgets inhibit the production of melatonin and push our body clocks later – another possible reason that you can wake up feeling groggy and tired. This is why I felt so exhausted for years, regardless of what supplements or night-time routines I used. If you're consistently waking up tired, it's probably the same thing that is happening to you. Thankfully, it's easy to address, which I'll come back to later. It's worth noting that the yellows, ambers and reds that illuminate from a fire don't affect melatonin, so light from fires and candles don't negatively affect your sleep the way blue light does. It's inevitable, though, that you're not always going to have a good night's sleep. What do you do then?

Mitigating a poor night's sleep

1. Caffeinate smart. Let's call a spade a spade. Caffeine is a drug. It's legal, it's widely available worldwide and it's absolutely wonderful, but it's still a drug. Thinking about it like this can allow you to use it as a potent tool, either in your workout arsenal or to mitigate the damage of a poor night's sleep. The temptation after a poor night's sleep is to load up on caffeine or stimulants to get through the following day, but I'd advise that you don't over-consume caffeine, regardless of how tired you feel. Despite the exhaustion you may feel from sleep deprivation, consuming too much caffeine may reduce the quality of the next night's sleep. One or two cups of coffee during the day – instead of 10 – will keep your eyes open without derailing your next night of sleep.

2. Move more. The best way to reset your internal clock is to get outside and get some sunshine and exercise. This can be some light aerobic exercise, or even a brisk walk. The movement, light and vitamin D will help to realign your circadian rhythm and eliminate some of your sleep-deprivation anxiety – that random edginess that accompanies a poor night's sleep. My tip is to not overthink it. Get up, get dressed, load up a music playlist or podcast and just go. You'll feel so much better throughout the entire day for it.

3. Eat right. Your sleep cycle regulates your appetite. When you are sleep deprived, your hunger hormone ghrelin levels will be high and your satiated hormone leptin will be low – I

explained both of these earlier in the book. The temptation is to reach for refined carbs, sugars and fats during this period, buts that's just going to make you feel even more tired. Your goal is achieving a slow and steady burn of energy. Look for foods that are high in protein, moderate in fat, and low on the glycaemic index. Protein intake can also increase the production of orexin, a hormone that keeps you awake and alert. This can work wonderfully well on days like this; but be mindful of your protein intake before bed, for the same reason. In my early bodybuilder days, I would eat two chicken breasts before bed and could never figure out why I would find myself staring at the ceiling for the night. It wasn't until I learnt about orexin, years later, that it all started to make sense to me.

4. Nap (if you need to). While there are certainly dangers that accompany regular polyphasic sleep – sleep in multiple shorter sessions, rather than in one large chunk – naps can definitely help you get through a brief period of sleep deprivation. When my daughter was born in 2015 and I was preparing for a fitness model competition, I found it impossible to get a solid seven or eight hours every night. At the time, I found that two 90-minute naps, and then three to four hours at night-time, got me through that period. I don't recommend it long term, but it is a good short-term strategy. I would strongly advise new parents, college students on study binges or anybody who has regularly broken sleep patterns at night-time to check out sleep expert Nick Littlehales's book, *Sleep*.

What's your chronotype?

When it comes to sleep research, my biggest personal fascination has been with chronotypes. Whether you stumble into bed before the sun goes up or rise with the roosters, most of us can identify with a specific sleep type or chronotype, even if we've never called it that. If you were like me, you were aware of it, but never actually knew what it was called. Let me ask you a question that will shed a light on this. Are you a night owl or a morning person? Chances are you have used that language at some point in your life. That's chronotypes explained in a nutshell. A night owl – somebody who prefers to rise and go to bed later – is one form of chronotype. A morning person – somebody who generally goes to bed and rises early – is another form of chronotype. It's basically a person's circadian typology, or the individual differences in activity and alertness in the morning and evening. 'Knowing your chronotype may help you understand how your internal clock works and how you can synchronize it with your daily activities and duties to use your time most efficiently,' explains certified sleep science coach Eva Cohen. In particular, Cohen says that your chronotype defines your peak productivity times, allowing you to plan your day wisely.

Most research breaks chronotypes into:
- Morning type
- Evening type
- Neither

Some describe four types, with the names:
- Bear
- Wolf

- Lion
- Dolphin

The bear

Most people fall under the category of a bear chronotype. This means their sleep and wake cycle goes according to the sun. Cohen says bear chronotypes wake easily and typically fall asleep with no problem. Productivity seems best before noon, and they're prone to a 'post-lunch dip' between 2 and 4 p.m. That post-lunch dip can generally be addressed with correct nutrition, but for chronotype purposes, it serves to illustrate the point.

The wolf

This chronotype often has trouble waking in the morning. In fact, Cohen says wolf chronotypes feel more energetic when they wake up at noon, especially since their peak productivity starts at noon and ends about four hours later. My videographer Tommy is exactly like this. Anytime I tell him we're shooting at 9 a.m. – I've normally been up for four hours at this point – I can see a little bit of his soul die inside. He's told me on several occasions that he does his best editing and work at around 1 a.m. This probably isn't ideal if you work nine to five in an office; but it's great awareness to have if you're self-employed, run your own business or have flexibility with your work schedule so that you can optimise your productivity. Wolf types tend to get another boost around 6 p.m. and find they can get a lot done while everyone else is finished for the day.

The lion

Unlike wolves, lion chronotypes like to rise early in the morning. 'They may easily wake up before dawn and are at their best up until noon,' says Cohen. Typically, lion types wind down in the evening and end up falling asleep by 9 or 10 p.m. As someone who goes to bed around 9 or 10 p.m. and gets up at 5 or 6 a.m., I fall right into this category.

The dolphin

If you have trouble following any sleep schedule, then you may be a dolphin. 'They often don't get enough sleep due to their sensitivity to different disturbing factors like noise and light,' says Cohen. The good news? Dolphins have a peak productivity window from 10 a.m. to 2 p.m., which is a great time to get things done.

Can you change your chronotype?

This is where the research and my own anecdotal opinion differ greatly. The current sleep research says that due to underlying biological and genetic factors, each person's chronotype is hard-coded. This means you can't physically change or alter your chronotype, as it's determined by the PER3 gene. Now, I'm not going to be 'that guy' and argue against gene research, as it's so far outside my circle of competence, it makes my head spin. However, for years I was a night owl, and although the research[20] suggests that your chronotype changes with age, my experience and the research don't match up.

In my early twenties, I would have to force myself to go to bed at around 10 p.m. in order to get up for work as a teacher the following day. At the weekends or during school holidays, I'd comfortably crawl into bed around 2 a.m. and sleep until about 10 a.m. the next day. Then in 2017, I joined what I call the '5 a.m. club' – I started getting up every morning (Monday to Friday) at 5 a.m. The reasons for this were mostly personal: my increased training volume meant that I had to work out for several hours each day in preparation for a race or event, but I didn't want that to affect my time with family, friends or even my work. It was horrible for about a year and a half. From 2017 to mid-2018, I would have to drag myself out of bed every single morning; I felt like I was fighting my biology and my natural urge to sleep later. Then, towards the back end of 2018, it got easier. Six months later, it even started to feel natural. Now there are some mornings where I wake up 10 or 15 minutes before my alarm at 5 a.m.

As I said, I'm not questioning the current research, as when offering advice, I generally like to have an evidence-backed approach – but sleep research is still in its infancy, so I feel okay sharing my experience. As someone who would never have claimed to be a morning person, I now firmly fall into that bracket. I bring this up because I was fortunate enough to have come across the research that says you can't change your chronotype only after I had successfully changed it. One of my mentors used to tell me the not very optimistic, but paradoxically inspiring line, 'The people who change the world were normally just too stupid to realise they couldn't', which basically means that they didn't listen to what the world or people said they could or couldn't do. I'm not saying that my individual experience that contradicts the research of people much smarter than me falls into that bracket; but I think that mindset is useful when approaching every study or research you read. Trust, but verify. If your personal experience doesn't align with what research says, be it in sleep, nutrition or anything we cover in this book, understand that individual variability is a real thing, and you are always going to be your own best example. As a former wolf who now finds himself claiming to be a lion, I like to think of myself as proof that you can change your chronotype. But then again, maybe there's a massive gap in my knowledge and I was always a lion parading around in wolf clothing. Who knows? Now that we've covered the basics of sleep, let's get on to how to improve your overall sleep quality. I'll start with the supplements.

SLEEP SUPPLEMENTS

For some, minimising blue light and caffeine or stimulants closer to bedtime is enough to get a great night's sleep. However, if you find yourself really needing a supercharge, there are some supplements that can work well by either helping you fall asleep or keeping you in a deeper sleep for longer. Always check your supplements to verify their compatibility with medications that you may be taking, as some vitamins and minerals have been known to reduce the effect of some medications, such as birth control pills. There are hundreds of sleep supplements on the market, but certain compounds are known to be more effective than others in improving sleep onset latency, wake times and deep sleep percentages. Below, I'll identify these and other nutrients that can help you maximise your sleep.

Zinc

This is an important supplement for male and female fertility and therefore for libido, as zinc deficiency can lead to lower testosterone levels. Both men and women need balanced testosterone levels for optimal hormonal support. Zinc can support testosterone production by putting you into a deeper sleep, which also improves recovery dramatically for individuals who work out or move a lot, as zinc is one of the first minerals to get depleted in gym-goers, athletes or anyone with high activity levels.

Dosage

It is normally best taken at a dosage of 25mg per day with magnesium (see below) and vitamin B6 (ZMA), about 30 minutes before bed on an empty stomach.

Magnesium

Unfortunately, at the time of writing, magnesium deficiency is incredibly common, and I include myself in that. Refined/processed foods are stripped of their mineral, vitamin and fibre content. These are anti-nutrient foods because they actually steal magnesium in order to be metabolised. If these food are consumed and not supplemented with magnesium, we become increasingly deficient. Are you tense and tight or crave chocolate? Anything that makes you tense or tight could be potentially due to a magnesium deficiency, which is one reason why you may crave chocolate at night-time or when stressed. Dark chocolate, especially, is one of the highest food sources of magnesium. The case of consuming chocolate is a catch-22 though. Even though it has magnesium, chocolate also has sugar. Every molecule of sugar you consume pulls over 50 times the amount of magnesium out of the body. Try and go for an 85 per cent or higher dark chocolate to minimise your daily sugar intake.

Dosage

Try taking 600–800mg a day 30 minutes before bed. However, be careful, as too much too soon can give you a stomach upset. When you get the correct dosage, due to its mild effect on your central nervous system, you can find that you are much more relaxed going to bed.

GABA

GABA is an inhibitory neurotransmitter that your brain uses to shut itself down. The GABA supplementation research is still a little inconclusive as to its overall effectiveness, but personally I like it a lot and use it regularly. I normally consume it 60 minutes after my meal or on an empty stomach. I find GABA great as a bedtime supplement, but also use it during the day if I'm feeling particularly stressed or anxious during busy work weeks.

Dosage

Start with 500mg before bed. This dosage can go as high as 2,500mg (incrementing the dose). GABA has also been shown to raise human growth hormone (HGH) in the higher end of dosage (discussed in the next pages).

L-theanine

The amino acid L-theanine is most commonly found in green tea leaves but can also be taken as a supplement. It can significantly reduce stress and increase relaxation without causing drowsiness, most notably when combined with a source of caffeine (such as an afternoon cup of coffee) that would normally disrupt sleep. Research[21] suggests that L-theanine crosses the blood-brain barrier in about 30 minutes and improves mental relaxation without loss of alertness by acting directly on the central nervous system. Once it crosses the blood-brain barrier, it reduces sympathetic nervous system activity, improves post-stress relaxation and reduces cortisol and anxiety.

Dosage

Start with a dose of 100 to 200mg. If you consume it with a caffeine source like coffee or a caffeine tablet, consume it at 1:4 caffeine to L-theanine ratio. For example, when I was running through the Arctic, I consumed 100mg of caffeine with 400mg of L-theanine three times a day, to help keep my energy levels high but balanced during the race. This also meant that I had no problem sleeping at night-time, even with caffeine in my system.

TWELVE TIPS FOR HEALTHY SLEEP

The science and logistics of sleep are incredibly important, and the host of tools, hacks and strategies for optimising sleep can be long and confusing; but I've tried to break them down into 12 tips below. This section was inspired by Matthew Walker's international bestseller *Why We Sleep,* which is a fascinating read for anyone interested in further educating themselves on the science of sleep.

1. **Stick to a sleep schedule.** Go to bed and wake up at the same time each day. As creatures of habit, people have a hard time adjusting to changes in sleep patterns. Sleeping later on the weekend won't fully make up for a lack of sleep during the week and will make it harder to wake up early on Monday morning. When I worked as a primary school teacher in London, I thought I could make up my sleep debt every weekend, but it just made me even more tired. I recommend setting an alarm for bedtime if you have to. In 2016, when I joined the 5 a.m. club, I used to set an alarm for 8:30 p.m. every evening to remind myself that I had to be in bed in half an hour. It worked really well, and after several weeks I didn't need to set an alarm anymore. Most people set an alarm for when it's time to wake up, but it's much less common to do so for when it's time to go to sleep. If you only take one piece of advice from this section, let it be this.

2. **Exercise is great, but not too late in the day.** Exercise releases cortisol and that works in opposition to melatonin. Try to exercise at least 30 minutes on most days – even if it's just hitting your daily step count – but not later than two or three hours before bed.

3. **Avoid or minimise caffeine and nicotine.** Coffee, cola, certain teas and some chocolates contain caffeine, and its effect can take as long as 11 hours to fully wear off. Therefore, a cup of coffee in the late afternoon can make it hard for you to fall asleep at night. Nicotine is also a stimulant, often causing smokers to sleep only very lightly. My old housemate and one

of my best friends, Niall, was a chronically poor sleeper until he gave up cigarettes; now he claims he sleeps like a baby every night. In addition, smokers can often wake up too early in the morning because of nicotine withdrawal.

4. **Avoid alcoholic drinks before bed.** Having a night cap or alcoholic beverage before sleep may help you relax, but heavy use robs you of REM sleep, keeping you in lighter stages of sleep throughout the night. You may also tend to wake up in the middle of the night when the effects of alcohol have worn off, something that happened to me regularly during my college days. I found I had to sleep extra-late the following morning, or nap just to get through the day.

5. **Avoid large meals or beverages late at night.** A light snack is okay and may even help certain people sleep, but a large meal can cause indigestion, which interferes with sleep. Drinking too many fluids at night, meanwhile, can cause frequent awakening to urinate – something I'm sure everyone has experienced at some stage.

6. **If possible, avoid medication that delays or disrupts your sleep.** This is straight from Matthew Walker's book. Some commonly prescribed heart, blood pressure or asthma medications, as well as some over-the-counter herbal remedies for coughs, colds or allergies, can disrupt sleep patterns. If you have trouble sleeping, talk to your healthcare provider or pharmacist to see whether any drugs you're taking might be contributing to your insomnia, and ask whether they can be taken at other times during the day or early in the evening.

7. **Don't nap after 3 p.m.** Naps can help make up for lost sleep, but late-afternoon naps can make it harder to fall asleep at

night. This obviously depends on what time of the day you go to bed. If I'm planning an early-morning workout at 5 a.m. and going to bed at 9 p.m., I can't generally nap any later than 12 p.m. that day. You may need to experiment with this, but 3 p.m. is a good cut-off point for an average bedtime.

8. **Relax before bed.** Don't overschedule your day so that there is no time left for unwinding. I normally switch my phone off and turn off work mode at around 6 p.m. every day, or 7 p.m. at the latest. This generally gives me an hour or two to unwind before bed, whether that's with family members, friends or otherwise. A relaxing activity, such as reading or listening to music, are good examples of a bedtime ritual.

9. **Take a hot bath before bed.** The drop in body temperature after getting out of the bath may help you feel sleepy, and the bath can help you relax and slow down so you're more ready to sleep. Personally, I like to add four or five cups of Epsom salts to a hot bath and then finish with 30 seconds in a cold shower. The cold shower is optional, of course, as some don't respond well to the cold; but for me, it's my favourite bedtime ritual on extra-stressful days or days of extremely difficult workouts.

10. **Dark bedroom, cool bedroom, gadget-free bedroom.** Get rid of anything in your bedroom that might distract you from sleep, such as noises, bright lights, an uncomfortable bed or warm temperatures. You sleep better if the temperature in the room is kept on the cool side. A TV, phone or computer in the bedroom can be a distraction and deprive you of needed sleep. I found removing the TV and laptop was pretty straightforward; but I use my phone for an alarm, so that was

more difficult. Now I set the alarm before bed and then put it on airplane mode so that I don't get distracted by it. Having a comfortable mattress and pillow can help promote a good night's sleep. Individuals with insomnia or a history of poor sleep often watch the clock. Turn the clock's face out of view so you don't worry about the time while trying to fall asleep. If you find yourself lying awake doing the dreaded 'If I fall asleep now, I'll get six hours of sleep', I recommend removing the clock from your room entirely.

11. **Have the right sunlight exposure.** Daylight is key to regulating daily sleep patterns. Try to get outside in natural sunlight for at least 30 minutes every day. If possible, wake up with the sun or use very bright lights in the morning. Sleep experts recommend that if you have problems falling asleep, you should get an hour of exposure to morning sunlight and turn down the lights before bedtime. I have bright light bulbs in all the rooms I enter in the morning – sitting room, kitchen, hallway – and have softer, orange-tinted lights in the room I spend the evening in: my bedroom, study and bedroom toilet. It's a small and easy hack that pays off massively with your sleep quality.

12. **Don't lie in bed awake**. If you find yourself still awake after staying in bed for more than 20 minutes, or if you are starting to feel anxious or worried, get up and do some relaxing activity until you feel sleepy. The anxiety of not being able to sleep can make it harder to fall asleep. I should recommend a book or some meditation but that's never worked for me. On the nights I find myself staring at the ceiling, I normally put on my blue-light-blocking glasses and turn on Sky Sports news

for the football updates. After 10 or 15 minutes, I normally find myself yawning and just go back to bed. That's not necessarily a recommendation (you might hate sports), but it is an example of finding what works best for you and then keeping that tool in your arsenal.

Now that we know how important sleep is for our weight, mood and wellbeing, let's look at the next potential pitfall that can negatively affect your progress. Although it's normally relegated to the back burner, I think it's about time it was elevated to its rightful position at the front of your mind. I'm talking about stress.

The facts about stress

What do we do know about stress? Apparently, not enough. People are highly aware of its adverse aspects, yet there is little known in popular culture about its beneficial role. Yes, beneficial. Understanding how stress can work for you is the key to managing your waistline, reducing anxiety and improving your overall quality of life. Before we dive deep into the pros and cons of stress, there is an important term that you need to be familiar with first: hormesis. Hormesis is a process of adaption: it makes stress work for you rather than against you. It's a basic adaptative stress response, which means that short bursts or low doses of something can make you stronger, more robust or better able to handle a larger stressor later on. Weightlifting or resistance training is an example of this. You lift weights, which triggers a stress response, your muscles repair and signal that you might need to be able to do that movement at X amount of weight again, so your body gets stronger to enable you to cope with it next time. Obviously, that's a ridiculously simplified and linear example of a much more complicated and nuanced physiological process, but it's pretty much that in a nutshell.

Another example I like to use to explain hormesis is tanning before a sun holiday. If you're fair skinned and likely to burn before you go on a sun holiday to Spain, it makes sense to get a base layer tan. Some will do this in their back garden; others with tanning beds – this isn't a recommendation, just an example of what people do. You expose yourself to a little bit of sun for 14 to 21 days before you go on holiday and then that base layer can prevent, or at least reduce, your risk of burning the first day of your holiday when you're sitting poolside with a piña colada in your hand. That's like the hormetic response. You expose yourself in a shortened and controlled setting (i.e. back-garden tanning) so you can handle a big stressor later (the sun heat of Spain). We'll come back to this later, but it's important to understand the hormetic process before we go any further. Now back to stress.

Picture this. You're sprinting down the street with a lion after you. Things looked grim for a moment there, but, luckily for you, your cardiovascular system kicked into gear, and now it's delivering oxygen and energy to your exercising muscles. But what energy? There's not enough time to eat a chocolate bar and derive its benefits as you sprint along; there's not even enough time to digest food already in your gut. Your body must get energy from its places of storage, like fat or stored glycogen that you got from your morning bowl of porridge and the rice you had at lunch a few hours ago. To understand how you mobilise energy in this scenario, and how that mobilisation can work against you at times, we need to understand how the body stores energy in the first place.

The basic process of digestion consists of breaking down the food we eat. We can't make use of the food exactly as it is – we can't, for example, make our back muscles stronger by grafting on the piece of turkey we ate. If only it were that easy. Instead, complex food matter is broken down into its simplest parts (molecules): amino acids, simple sugars like glucose and free fatty acids; all of which we touched on in an earlier section about macro nutrients. A table in Robert Sapolsky's book on stress, *Why Zebras Don't Get Ulcers*, illustrates it better than I could, but here's a simplified version.

What you stick in your mouth	Protein	Starch, sugars, carbo-hydrates	Fat
How it winds up in your blood stream	Amino acids	Glucose	Fatty acids and glycerol
How it gets stored if you have a surplus	Protein	Glycogen	Triglycerides
How it gets mobilised in stressful emergencies	Amino acids	Glucose	Fatty acids, glycerol, ketone bodies

Excess protein consumed is usually stored as fat, while the surplus of amino acids is excreted. This can lead to weight gain over time, especially if you consume too many calories while trying to increase your protein intake.

This strategy of breaking your food down into its simplest parts and reconverting it into complex storage forms is precisely what your body should do when you've eaten plenty. And it is precisely what your body should *not* do in the face of an immediate physical emergency. Then, you want to stop energy storage. Turn up the activity of the sympathetic nervous system (fight or flight response), turn down the parasympathetic (rest and digest), and down goes insulin secretion. Thousands of years ago, that stress response potentially saved your ancestors from being eaten by a lion in the African savannah, but that exact scenario is less likely to happen on your commute to the office on a Wednesday. But your basic physiology hasn't changed much since then. Replace 'chased by a lion' with 'shouted at by your boss', 'demeaned by your other half' or 'made fun of by a friend or in a social setting', and that stress response is nearly identical. But what has that got to do with weight loss? Actually, a lot.

CORTISOL – THE STRESS HORMONE

Think of cortisol as nature's built-in alarm system. It's your body's main stress hormone, and it works with certain parts of your brain to control your mood, motivation and fear. Your adrenal glands – triangle-shaped organs at the top of your kidneys – make cortisol. It's best known for helping fuel your body's 'fight or flight' instinct in a crisis, but cortisol plays an important role in a number of things your body does. For example, it:

- Manages how your body uses carbohydrates, fats and proteins.
- Keeps inflammation down.
- Regulates your blood sugar.
- Increases your blood sugar (glucose).
- Controls your sleep/wake cycle – it's the daily rise in cortisol that helps you wake up every day. I like to think of melatonin (aka the sleep hormone) as the opposite to cortisol. Melatonin released from your pituitary gland helps you wind down at night to prepare for sleep and cortisol helps you wake up. There's more on this in the preceding sleep chapter.
- Boosts energy so you can handle stress and restores balance afterwards. Think of the example of the lion above.

But how does it work? Your hypothalamus and pituitary gland – both located in your brain – can sense if your blood contains the right level of cortisol. If the level is too low, your brain adjusts the amount of hormones it makes. Your adrenal glands pick up on these signals. Then they fine-tune the amount of cortisol they release.

Cortisol receptors – which are in most cells in your body – receive and use the hormone in different ways. Your needs will differ from day to day. For instance, when your body is on high alert, cortisol can alter or shut down functions that get in the way. These might include your digestive or reproductive systems (aka your sex drive), your immune system or even your lipolytic processes (aka burning fat). Sometimes, your cortisol can get out of whack, which leads to a whole host of problems.

Too much stress

After the pressure or danger has passed, your cortisol level should calm down, bringing your heart, blood pressure and other body systems back to normal. But what if you're under constant stress and the alarm button stays on? It can derail your body's most important functions. It can also lead to a number of health problems, including:

- Anxiety and depression
- Headaches
- Heart disease
- Memory and concentration problems
- Problems with digestion
- Trouble sleeping
- Our primary concern here – fat gain.

Too much cortisol

Too much cortisol and fat reduction doesn't make fat loss impossible, but it does make it considerably harder. It's kind of like climbing a hill. That in and of itself is demanding enough, as is fat loss, but having too much cortisol is like climbing the hill with an 18-kilo vest on. When it comes to reducing cortisol for fat loss, the stress management techniques later on in the chapter will help to keep them in check.

Too little cortisol

This is pretty rare, but as it happens from time to time, I want to touch on it here. If your body doesn't make enough of this hormone, you're likely have a condition doctors call Addison's disease. Usually, the symptoms appear over time. They include:

- Changes in your skin, like darkening on scars and in skin folds
- Being tired all the time
- Muscle weakness that grows worse
- Diarrhoea, nausea and vomiting
- Loss of appetite and weight
- Low blood pressure

This is outside the scope of this book; but if you think your body isn't making enough cortisol, I recommend you consult your doctor for a test.

Cortisol and weight loss

Researchers have long known that rises in stress and cortisol lead to weight gain. Every time you're stressed, your adrenal glands release adrenaline and cortisol and, as a result, glucose (your primary source of energy) is released into your bloodstream. All of this is done to give you the energy you need to escape from a risky situation. Once the threat has subsided, your adrenaline high wears off and your blood sugar spike drops. This is when cortisol kicks into high gear to replenish your energy supply quickly. If you've ever had an incredibly stressful day at work or in a relationship and completely forgotten to eat all day (cortisol inhibiting your digestive system), then arrive home at 6 p.m., realised you're starving and devoured an entire pizza or tub of ice-cream, you've experienced this stress response, even if you were unaware of it.

I remember when I was studying to become a primary school teacher back in 2010, any day I had a presentation or an observation for teaching practices, I would have knots in my stomach all day and could never eat more than a couple of rice cakes or a bite or two of chicken. As soon as the observation or presentation was finished, I'd have this cortisol dump and I'd rush to the shop to get as much chocolate, ice-cream or sugar I could get my hands on. Again, as you know by this stage, I'm not saying to avoid these foods; but stress-induced food or sugar cravings can be avoided if you're aware of them. Not managing them, or worse, being unaware of them and then trying to do damage limitation by starving yourself the following day is not only detrimental to your long-term weight-loss goals, but completely ruins your relationship with food in the process.

Cortisol and metabolism

Even if you aren't eating foods high in fat and sugar, cortisol can still slow down your metabolism, making it difficult to lose weight. In 2015, researchers from Ohio State University interviewed women about the stress they had experienced the previous day before feeding them a high-fat, high-calorie meal. After the women finished their meal, scientists measured the metabolic rate (the rate at which they burnt calories and fat) of each participant and examined their blood sugar, cholesterol, insulin and cortisol levels.

The researchers found that, on average, women who reported one or more stressors during the prior 24 hours burnt 104 fewer calories than non-stressed women.[22] All other things equal, this could potentially result in a five-kilo weight gain in one year.

Stressed individuals also have higher insulin levels, a hormone that contributes to fat storage.

STRESS-INDUCED UNHEALTHY HABITS

In addition to hormonal changes, stress can also drive you to engage in the following unhealthy behaviours, all of which can cause weight gain:

- Emotional eating: Increased levels of cortisol can not only make you crave unhealthy food, but excess nervous energy can often cause you to eat more than you normally would. You might find that snacking or reaching for a second helping provides you with some temporary relief from your stress but makes healthy weight management more difficult. See more on emotional eating in Part Two.

- Eating 'accessible' or fast food: When we are stressed, and not planning, we tend to eat the first thing we see and/or what is readily available and accessible, which is not always the healthiest option. You may also be more likely to drive to a fast-food place, rather than taking the time and mental energy to cook a balanced, healthy meal.

- Exercising less: With all the demands on your schedule, exercising may be one of the last things on your to-do list. Ironically, the hormetic response of short bursts of exercise can actually *lower* your overall cortisol levels; more on this later.

- Skipping meals: When you are juggling a dozen things at once, eating a healthy meal or food on your nutritional plan can drop down in the list of priorities. You might find yourself skipping breakfast because you're running late or not eating lunch because you're just too busy. Again, skipping breakfast can potentially be a useful tool on a fat loss plan (see the intermittent fasting section on p181), but there's a big difference between a plan with a scheduled intermittent fast that fits in with your lifestyle and schedule, and rushing out the door because your stress levels are jacked up to the nines. *Why* you do something can be just as important as what you do.

- Sleeping less: Many people report trouble sleeping when they're stressed, and research has linked sleep deprivation to a slower metabolism. Feeling overtired can also reduce willpower and contribute to unhealthy eating habits. Read more on this in the chapter on sleep.

HOW TO BREAK THE CYCLE OF STRESS AND WEIGHT GAIN

When you're stressed out, healthy behaviours such as eating properly and exercising regularly can easily fall by the wayside. Maintaining a schedule and/or routine can help make these healthy behaviours a habit and combat stress-related weight changes. Here are a few strategies that can help you break the cycle of stress and weight gain:

- Make exercise a priority. Exercising is a critical component of stress reduction and weight management. It can help you address both issues simultaneously, so it's essential for warding off stress-related weight gain. Whether it's going for a walk during your lunch break, taking a yoga class or hitting the gym after work, incorporate regular exercise into your routine.
- Eat healthier comfort foods. You don't need an excess of carbs or fats to make you feel better. One of the few studies testing

the effectiveness of comfort foods in improving mood found that eating relatively healthier comfort foods, such as low-calorie air-popped popcorn, is just as likely to boost a negative mood as the unhealthier alternatives – such as popcorn loaded with butter and salt.

- Practice mindful eating. Focusing on what you're eating without distractions may help lower stress, promote weight loss and prevent weight gain. This is heavily linked with emotional eating, which we've already talked about. One study[23] found that overweight women who had mindfulness-based stress and nutrition training were better able to avoid emotional eating, and had lower stress levels, which led to less belly fat over time. Next time you eat a meal, try enjoying it without the distraction of your phone or the TV.

- Keep a food journal. Paying attention to your eating habits can help you gain control over your food consumption. A 2011 review of studies that examined the link between self-monitoring and weight loss found that those who kept a food journal were more likely to manage their weight than those who didn't.[24] So, whether you use an app like MyFitnessPal to track your food intake or write everything in a food diary, being more mindful of what you put in your mouth could improve your eating habits. It's also useful to make note of the days you are feeling especially stressed and how your eating pattern or caloric intake changes as a result. A 1–10 scale, 1 being not stressed at all, 10 being wired to moon, works well.

- Drink more water. It's easy to confuse thirst for hunger, but mixing up these two cravings can lead you to eat more calories than your body needs, prompting weight gain. It's much easier to identify hunger after you've eliminated any mild dehydration. If it's only been a couple of hours since you've eaten and you feel hungry, try drinking some water first. If you still feel hungry, then grab a snack.

Now let's look at the other important areas when it comes to stress and your overall life quality: your sex drive and immune system.

STRESS AND YOUR SEX DRIVE

As a general rule, stress has been shown to reduce sexual performance or even destroy it completely. That's generally due to the inhibitory effect cortisol has on sex hormones. In a lot of cases, chronically poor dietary choices, long-term stress at work or just too much exercise can all negatively impact your sex drive. Funnily enough, as you'll see shortly, acute stressors such as cold exposure tend to have the opposite impact and can improve or increase your sex drive. Stress and sex are literally cross wired in your brain. The brain centre that controls the stress response, the HPA axis, shares hormones with the centre that controls sex, the hypothalamic-pituitary gonadal axis. That shows that the release of stress hormones is regulated with that of sex hormones. Hormesis, which we talked about at the start of the chapter, is a key determining factor here. Hormesis causes stress hormones to act like anti-stress hormones and boost the release of sex hormones; lack of hormesis causes stress hormones to inhibit sex hormones. Simply put, the acute stressors listed later on all positively impact your sex drive, and their absence negatively impacts it.

STRESS AND YOUR IMMUNE SYSTEM

As I'm sure you know, the primary job of the immune system is to defend the body against infectious agents such as viruses, bacteria, fungi and parasites. The immune system and its process is incredibly complex, and its intricacies are far beyond what I can cover in this book. Yet it's still worth understanding the connection between stress, your immune system and your ability to lose fat. If you're under the weather, have a cold or flu or are just generally sick, then it's significantly more difficult to adhere to any nutritional plan while your unwell body craves more comfort food until you're back to full health. Combine this with the reduction in movement that tends to come alongside sickness and you have a recipe for stalled fat loss, or fat gain if it's happening frequently, i.e. if you are sick at least once a month and the poor behavioural patterns are negatively compounding month on month.

Stress will suppress the formation of new lymphocytes (lymphocytes and monocytes are collectively known as white blood cells; cyte is a term for cells) and stalls their release into circulation, all the while shortening the time pre-existing lymphocytes stay in your body's circulation. Think of your white blood cells as your army that prevents you from getting sick. The viruses or bacteria, etc. are the invaders. As long as your white blood cells are strong and well equipped (through low stress, good nutrition and high-quality sleep), they will fight off most potential invaders. However, add chronic stress to the mix and your well-tuned army turn into a pile of snivelling weaklings without a weapon between them. Now you're increasingly at risk of getting sick. Again, the solution, as with stress and your sex drive above, is the same: include acute stressors and manage or reduce chronic stressors.

STRESS MANAGEMENT TECHNIQUES

When it comes to stress management techniques, perhaps the best way to begin is by making a mental list of the sorts of things we find stressful. No doubt you would immediately come up with some obvious examples – traffic, deadlines, family relationships, money worries, etc. If I left you long enough, it would start to transcend into the personal – a dislike for your current physical appearance, a nasty fight you had with your other half last night or a presentation you have at work tomorrow.

As mentioned earlier, we are thankfully no longer fearful of running away from a predatory lion – but that still doesn't stop our body responding in the exact same way to psychological or social disruptions. Regardless of how poorly we are getting along with a family member or how incensed we are about being cut off in traffic, we rarely settle that sort of thing in a fist fight and nowadays we have fewer places, or worse, have no idea how to channel that energy. It's the first law of thermodynamics – energy is never lost, it's only transferred – so if we don't find a way to manage or channel that stress, then it can cause a whole host of health problems. Not to mention making fat loss considerably more difficult.

Essentially, we humans live well enough and long enough, and are smart enough (if you want to call it that) to generate all sorts of stressful events purely in our heads. I spoke about the psychological impact of how you frame situations in my last book, *Rewire Your Mindset*; but viewed from the perspective of the evolution of the animal kingdom, sustained physiological stress is a recent invention, mostly limited to humans. Therefore, until our physiology has had the thousands of years (a low estimate) to catch up with new life-induced stressors, we're left with taking it back into our own hands with our stress management techniques.

We now know that not all stress is created equal. Acute or short-term stressors are actually very good for us; it's the chronic or long-term stress that wreaks havoc on your waistline and health. Shortly you'll see why you should expect stress to come along with reward. Lack of food makes food taste better; excessive heat makes cold feel good (and vice versa); and exercise brings relaxation. Biologically, we are programmed for compensations after stress, but if there's no reward, it's likely that you're veering towards chronic stress. In which case, I recommend a combination of acute stressors listed below.

Good stress
Short bursts of exercise

If you have ever had the good or relaxed feeling that follows exercise, then this will be nothing new to you, but how exactly does exercise reduce stress? Exercise is a form of physical stress and is just as important for your head and mental wellbeing as it is for your heart and overall health. If you've never followed a routine exercise regimen, then you may not agree with that at first; indeed, the first steps are the hardest, and in the beginning, exercise will be more work than fun. But as you get into shape, you'll begin to tolerate exercise, then enjoy it, and finally depend on it as a natural stress reliever. I don't think I've ever met a single person who enjoyed exercise when they first started, although lots of people forget how much they disliked it at first until they've crossed the chasm on the enjoyment scale. It's easy to misremember how you felt when you started to work out first, but I can recall it, and it sucked! It's hard, it makes you sore and it can be highly uncomfortable. But there is a 'tipping point' with it and at some point, you start to rewire or reframe all those associations as a positive thing when you get the relaxation or stress-free feeling that comes alongside exercise.

Regular exercise can bring remarkable changes to your body, your metabolism, your heart and your spirits. It has a unique capacity to exhilarate and relax, to provide stimulation and calm, to counter environmental depression (when life circumstances are getting you down) and to dissipate stress. It's a common experience among endurance athletes and has been verified in clinical trials[25] that have successfully used exercise to treat anxiety disorders and clinical depression. If athletes and patients can derive psychological benefits from exercise, so can you.

As someone who has a history of both environmental depression, from making really poor life choices in my early life, and crippling anxiety that led to panic attacks in my twenties, I was deeply interested in how exercise can contend with problems as difficult as anxiety and depression. There are several explanations, some chemical, others behavioural. The mental benefits of exercise have a neurochemical basis. Exercise reduces levels of the body's stress hormones, such as adrenaline and cortisol, which we've already touched on. It also stimulates the production of endorphins, chemicals in the brain that are the body's natural painkillers and mood elevators. Endorphins are responsible for the 'runner's high' and for the feelings of relaxation and optimism that accompany many hard workouts.

Behavioural factors also contribute to the emotional benefits of exercise. As your body fat reduces and your strength and stamina increase, your self-image can improve. You'll earn a sense of mastery and control, of pride and self-confidence. Your renewed vigour and energy will help you succeed in many tasks, and the discipline of regular exercise will help you achieve other important lifestyle goals. My morning workout is the foundation pillar upon which I build every day. Whether it's a 5km run, an intense leg workout or a brisk 40-minute walk, it anchors my day and keeps my mind clear for the day ahead.

Almost any type of exercise mentioned in the training section of this book will help. Many people find that using large muscle groups in a rhythmic, repetitive fashion works best, calling it 'muscular meditation,' and you'll begin to understand how it works. Walking and jogging are prime examples. Even a simple 20-minute stroll can clear the mind and reduce stress. But some people prefer vigorous workouts that burn stress along with calories. That's one reason why CrossFit is so popular. And the same stretching exercises that help relax your muscles after a hard workout will help relax your mind as well. The take-home message is that if you're looking to relieve stress, do some exercise. I recommend you experiment and find what you enjoy. If you currently dislike working out – and you're not alone if you do – try and habit stack with something social: join a running or hiking club, play five-a-side football or basketball, grab a friend and play tennis; if you can find exercise that doesn't really feel like exercise, then you're really on to a winner.

Cold exposure

Now I know what you're thinking: 'Cold, I hate the cold!' – and yours would be among the 99 per cent of responses I get when I mention cold exposure for stress relief. However, like exercise, cold exposure not only supports mental wellbeing but can potentially support fat loss too. This is due to the increased levels of BAT (brown adipose tissue) in populations who are regularly exposed to cold; but the research is still ongoing in this area, so I'll keep the focus on cold exposure and stress relief for now.

For me, I started to go deep on the research with cold exposure when I was preparing to run through the Arctic in 2019. Like most people, I had a severe aversion to the cold; but as I started to look into the research and, more importantly, apply it in my preparation for the Arctic, I found that it was like nothing else in terms of short-term benefit with very little exposure. What I mean by that is that I noticed the positive effects after as little as one minute a day of cold exposure! Sounds crazy, but hear me out. Research[26] shows that cold showers can potentially help with depression. After incorporating cold exposure into my everyday life for the three months prior to travelling to the Arctic Circle and seeing a huge reduction in my overall anxiety levels, I've experienced the link first-hand.

Cold showers have been proven to help improve blood circulation. When you cool down your body temperature, your system responds by moving fresh blood. Anxiety may cause an increase in blood pressure, so in theory, a cold shower may help bring it down. Another way cold showers may work is by increasing endorphins in your brain, similar to the 'runner's high' mentioned earlier. Endorphins can ease symptoms of depression and anxiety. Cold water may also decrease cortisol, the stress-inducing hormone we've focused on earlier in the chapter. Athletes have long been known to use ice baths to help decrease the inflammation that may lead to muscle soreness after an intense workout. For anxiety, a cold shower may reap similar benefits in terms of inflammation. Ongoing stress may increase inflammation, which can then lead to a cycle of inflammation-induced anxiety. Also, a cold shower can temporarily take your mind off the things you might be worried or fearful of. The minutes you spend focused on how the cold water feels on your body may act as a mindfulness practice, keeping you in the moment versus future events that are out of your control. Which begs the question, how do I get started?

When it comes to cold exposure for beginners, I think the Wim Hof Protocol is best. Wim Hof holds multiple world records for cold exposure and is the author of the book *The Wim Hof Method*. In the book, he explains that 'going into the ice water can be quite shocking, so you'd better prepare your body if you want to try it'. But how do we do that? Most of us who live in the West take showers every day, and most of those are warm or hot showers, because we don't like the cold. But if you end your warm or hot shower with just 30 seconds of cold water – just 30 seconds – you will begin to see results.

Anybody can endure 30 seconds of cold water, especially after spending several minutes under the warm or hot water; then you can increase that over time if you decide to. My advice is to start slowly in the beginning, with just 15 seconds at the end of your normal shower. Then a week later, go to 30 seconds, a week after that, 45 seconds and finally a full one to two minutes at the end of your normal shower. You'll notice the anti-anxiety effects pretty quickly and may even get a little bit addicted and transition to ice baths or cryotherapy over the coming months. Either way, building up to one to two minutes at the end of your normal shower can reap huge benefits. Be prepared – it's extremely uncomfortable at first as your body improves on its natural 'gasp or shiver' response, but by the end of the month you'll hardly be shivering, if at all. If you have a history of mental health problems, I'll even bet that you will start to look forward to the final minute of your daily shower. It's a potent tool for stress relief, but ease in slowly and build up gradually to avoid any potential complications. If you live close to the sea, you could also try a morning dip or sea swim – just be careful of how long you expose yourself to the cold based on the time of year. It's going to be considerably colder during the winter than in the summer months, so as with the cold showers, start with 30 seconds and increase exposure time gradually.

Heat exposure

This was another area of stress relief that I stumbled into by accident. When I was preparing to run through the Sahara in 2018, I was checking out the literature for heat exposure and came across some very interesting findings. At the time, there was a lot of anecdotal evidence about using heat (dry sauna mainly) and its positive impact on mood. Truthfully, I didn't think too much about it – I was looking for ways to improve my overall time in the sauna to withstand the 40–50 degree heat in the Sahara – but similar to the cold exposure above, I noticed a very peculiar, albeit incredible benefit from my exposure to heat.

Any day I did 20 minutes or more in the sauna, my perceived level of stress was greatly reduced for several hours after. Since 2018, there has been more and more research[27] for the impacts of sauna on heat-shock proteins, brain-derived neurotropic factor and most importantly, reduced levels of cortisol. Similar to the cold exposure discussed previously, I recommend experimenting with it yourself and seeing how you feel.

As with exercise and the cold, heat from the sauna relaxes the body's muscles, improves circulation and stimulates the release of endorphins. If your gym or local pool has a sauna, try 10–20 minutes after your workout. If it's an infrared sauna, you will probably need to double or treble your time inside to elicit a similar response to a wet steam sauna. You're looking to get to a level that's clearly uncomfortable but long before any risk of passing out, so proceed with caution, as heat tolerance varies greatly from person to person. If you don't have access to a sauna, try 10–20 minutes in a hot bath instead. If your body is sore from workouts, try adding three or four cups of Epsom salts to further enhance recovery.

Fasting

I've already discussed fasting in relation to weight loss or fat loss, but the research is quite strong on it as a hormetic stressor,[28] so I wanted to include it here also. Again, the duration of the fast can be as little as 12 hours to upwards of multiple days. Although I'm not a big fan of prolonged fasting as a long-term strategy for weight or fat loss – due to obvious adherence issues with a lack of food – I quite like it as a tool for an acute stress response.

Bad stress

'Bad' stress can come in lots of shapes and forms, but I've tried to condense them into the ones I most commonly see with people I work with.

Unhappy with a relationship (romantic, family, friend or otherwise)

I'm not going to dive into the first two examples in too much detail here as they were the focus of my last book, *Rewire Your Mindset*, but what I can say is that if you are unhappy with any relationship in your life, you are generally the only one who can change it. You might need to have an uncomfortable conversation or an awkward encounter, but that short-term pain generally leads to long-term gain, especially when it comes to your stress levels, mental health and wellbeing.

An unfulfilling job that makes you miserable

Tell me what you do every day and I'll tell you where you'll be in a year. I used this quote earlier about your nutrition and exercise programme, but it's even more applicable to your job. If you go to a location every day, or five days of the week, and that place makes you miserable, I can nearly guarantee you won't be maximising your happiness over the coming 12 months. Low happiness perceptions generally lead to increased stress levels, so you may need to get to the root of the cause if you're feeling unhappy or unfulfilled. As with the example above, nobody is going to improve your situation but you. Like every change I've mentioned in this book, you don't have to do it now or make drastic changes overnight, but if your ladder is against the wrong wall when it comes to your job, it's probably worth looking at getting it up against the right wall at some stage soon.

Poor nutrition

Too much salt, sugar or trans fats can wreak havoc on your stress levels. We have covered the downsides of all of these already; and thankfully the nutritional plan in this book should serve to cover that area for us.

Too much exercise (especially cardio)

This is where I want go deep, as it may be the area that you have the most misinformation around. Now, I can't really talk here. I regularly train for multiple hours a day and run ultra-marathons and compete in triathlons, but this is the one section in the book where I'm going to tell you: *Do as I say but not as I do.* On top of destabilising your digestion and your gut microbiome, too much exercise can increase the systemic circulation of cortisol in your body.

Research also shows prolonged cardio – logging runs over 10km, for example – can be an ineffective means to lose weight. By up-regulating cortisol, cardio can have the complete opposite effect of what you're trying to accomplish – it can actually contribute to your body holding on to the kind of 'stubborn fat' so many people have trouble losing. We discussed this in Part One.

The main issue here is that prolonged cardio breaks down muscle tissue rather than building it. This is why long-term marathon runners often look thin, saggy, and have an exaggerated kyphotic curve, i.e. an exaggerated, forward rounding of the back. They've amassed thousands of hours of training but never developed any muscle while doing it. The other issue with excessive cardio is its link with chronic joint damage. The repetitive impact caused by long-distance running, for example, puts stress on the joints and compromises joint positions. Combine this with an inadequate recovery protocol or not giving the body enough time to recover between workouts, and it all adds up. If you've got a running background and your goal is to run a marathon someday, this may sound like a knock back, and unfortunately, there's research that backs it up. When comparing a quadriceps biopsy (a biopsy is a sample of tissue taken from the body in order to examine it more closely) of a distance runner with a sprinter's, the marathoner's muscle shows significant cell damage, whereas the sprinter's does not.

As in most cases with this book, context is key. If you want to be a long-distance runner or bike the Tour de France, by all means, do it. I do, but I partake in these activities for the adventure and challenge, not for body compositional change. I also realise that this is not the optimal path if your aim is to be healthier and thinner, with any significant muscle development or definition. Although I stay on top of my strength training, I'm aware my excess cardio may actually be counterproductive to achieving any body composition goals. That's why context is key. If my goal was weight loss and body composition, I'd be focusing on my fat loss pyramid of prioritisation and nutrition. At the time of writing, those are not my personal fitness goals (although working specifically with individuals in that bracket is), but I wanted to give context as to what I recommend versus what I actually do.

If you happen to be similar to me and you engage on long bouts of cardiovascular activity for a different reason other than fat loss (a challenge, fun, adventure, etc.), but you have a secondary goal of body composition, I recommend you put a big focus on finding a nutritional plan that works for you; not dissimilar to the message preached throughout the entire book, but adjust your calories, carbohydrates or fats accordingly to match to your daily exercise needs. Personally, from a cortisol standpoint, I also try to take two to three months off heavy training after each extra-long endurance event that I do, in order to let my physiology return to normal. During this time, I normally go back to training four or five days a week with 40-to-50-minute workouts: usually some HIIT sessions, hypertrophy workouts or some form of CrossFit. Ultra-marathon and ironman medals are great, but if they come at the expense of my energy levels, my libido or immune system, then it's just not worth the trade-off, in my opinion.

THE LAST WORD ON STRESS

The quote 'knowledge is power', normally attributed to Sir Francis Bacon, really summarises stress. For too long, I only thought of stress as a 'bad' thing, and although I intrinsically knew that things like exercise made me feel good, I didn't really have anything to back that up apart from personal experience. I also had large gaps in my knowledge around hormesis, and the profound impact on the biological markers from exposure to acute stressors like heat and cold. Stress really is a double-edged sword that reminds me of Goldilocks and the three bears. Goldilocks found one bowl of porridge too cold, one too hot and one just right. It was the same with the beds: one was too hard, another too soft and the third just right. Stress is the same. Too little, and it causes a whole host of problems; too much and the issues are even worse. However, with just the right amount of stress in the shape of exercise, cold and/or heat exposure, you'll find yourself echoing the words of our Goldilocks herself: 'This is just right.'

Part Five
The Plan and Recipes

How to build your own nutritional plan

If you've been reading this book in a linear order, you know that your mindset and the way your approach your nutrition is going to play a much larger role in your success than the actual diet plan you follow. However, with that in mind, I will give you some best practices, recipes and an actual sample nutritional plan that you can implement straight away. I wouldn't look at this as a literal 'This is exactly how you need to eat from this point onwards', but as a guide that can get you from 0 to 1, following which you can course-correct as you go along. When it comes to building your own plan, it requires a bit of trial and error. It's also worth considering that you need to take your personal preferences, medical history and lifestyle factors into account.

For a weight-loss plan, I like to keep things simple. The focus is on getting a good-quality breakfast, lunch and dinner, and then adding in healthy snacks as required. Part One of the book goes through how you can do all your calorie calculations, but if that still confuses you, the good news is that you may not even need to do that. If you're incorporating these recipes, adding an exercise option from the last section and rewiring your mindset, you will probably get away without doing any of the calculations. To lose body fat, you need to be in a calorie deficit, but testing how you feel and how your body is changing is better than any calculation tool.

I recommend trying this plan for seven to ten days and checking how your body is responding. If your body fat is reducing, then keep going as you are. However, if you want faster results, calculate your TDEE (explained in Part One), track your calories for a few days, and make sure you are in a calorie deficit.

	Monday	Tuesday	Wednesday	Thursday	Friday	Saturday	Sunday
Breakfast 7 a.m.	Strawberry Greek yoghurt pancakes	Spiced scrambled eggs with smoked salmon and asparagus	Shakshuka	Blueberry and almond butter protein porridge	Pear baked oats	Simple homemade granola	Energy shake
Snack 10 a.m.	Coconut berry smoothie	Cashew and raisin oat bars	Chicken skewers with Greek yoghurt dip	Avocado toast with cottage cheese	Veggie chilli stuffed sweet potatoes	No snack	No snack
Lunch 1 p.m.	Salmon kebabs	Butternut squash soup	Sweetcorn fritters with fried egg and homemade salsa	Mediterranean chopped salad with mackerel and cucumber	Zingy chicken salad and wholewheat pitta	Red pepper and feta protein muffins	Slow cooker spicy chicken soup
Snack 4 p.m.	Piece of fruit	Handful of nuts	Piece of fruit	Handful of nuts	Piece of fruit	No snack	No snack
Dinner 7 p.m.	Sweet potato chicken curry with quinoa	Slow cooker chilli con carne with brown rice	Roasted curry salmon and brown rice	Baked falafel burgers and homemade chips	Garlic and herb roasted chicken and vegetables	Free meal	Steak with baby potatoes and homemade coleslaw

This is a very basic sample layout for your week; you can swap recipes, snacks and timings to fit your lifestyle and schedule. This entire book is built upon the philosophy of finding what works best for you. Although I was hesitant to include a sample meal plan at the risk of contradicting that message, this should serve as a visual for how your week might look, or – for those who are feeling motivated – offers a 'one and done' plan that you can follow straight away. The reason for the reduced snacks at the weekend is to balance out the calories from your weekly free meal (which can be whatever you want).

As stated above, I'd recommend testing this sample layout for seven to ten days. If your body fat is reducing, keep going as is. If it's not, calculate your calories for the following week and see if you're actually in a calorie deficit. Then adjust your portion sizes or snacks accordingly. Retest your body fat levels after another seven to ten days, and if you get the desired response, continue with that. If not, consider dropping calories slightly more for the next week, until you get to the point where your body fat is reducing and you feel full, satiated and energised throughout the day. It will take a bit of trial and error, as no two bodies are identical, but if you're consistent with this approach, not only will it work now, it will work over the long term too.

Maintaining the Keane Edge

We started our journey together talking about baking a cake and the importance of having the ingredients to give yourself the Keane Edge. Education is important, but knowing what to do isn't enough. If that were the case, there wouldn't be thousands of diet and nutrition books out there. I wrote this book because I would see people making the same mistakes over and over again: jumping from one diet to the next or one trainer to another, never looking at the bigger picture, unable to see the wood for the trees! Although I've tried to break down many of the myths and misconceptions of the weight loss world, the reality is that you have to experiment for yourself and find what works best for you. I'm aware that it's easier to write a book that just tells you to do 'X, Y and Z', like so many diet books have done in the past – but what then? You do X, Y and Z for six weeks, lose some weight … and what happens after? I wrote this book so that that never happens to you again.

You know now how important the context is. We've broken down unsupportive beliefs around foods, we've gone deep on recovering from slip-ups and pressing the f*ck it button too often – but having all that knowledge and information is just the first step of the ladder. My goal with this book is to help you finally get your ladder up against the right nutritional wall and start climbing it. You're not going to wait until next Monday to get started: you're feeling motivated now, so start now! You're also not going to beat yourself up if you fall off track a few times – remember that failure is feedback. Identify what caused you to go off track and be mindful of it next time. But, most importantly, it's now time to take action. If you want to lose weight and get into the best shape of your life, you can – but you have to do the work. It's back to that cake-baking; knowing the exact recipe and what ingredients to use is all well and good, but it doesn't get you a cake. You actually have to mix everything together, put it in the oven, have patience and soon you'll have a beautiful and tasty cake. That doesn't happen instantly, and nor does getting the body you want. It takes time – but everything worth having takes time.

A Chinese proverb maintains that 'the best time to plant a tree was 20 years ago. The next best time is today'. Now is your time to start. Time is going to pass whether you want it to or not, so you may as well get your ladder up against the right wall and start climbing. Ask what would your 'target self' do, right now? What would be their next step? Even the longest journey starts with the first steps, so take your first step today. This book has given you the Keane Edge, and now all you have to do is apply it.

The recipes

Breakfast

As I've mentioned before, when weight loss is a goal, I recommend starting the day off with a nutritionally dense meal (unless, of course, you're following an intermittent fasting protocol – in which case you can skip straight to the lunch recipes). As with all the recipes coming up, it's about experimenting with which ones you like the most. Personally, I could happily eat the blueberry, almond butter and protein porridge every single morning, but you can prioritise your own preferences in your nutrition.

STRAWBERRY GREEK YOGHURT PANCAKES

Serves:	2	Protein (g):	23
Serving:	271g	Fat (g):	13
Calories (kcal):	415	Fibre (g):	8.3
Carbs (g):	47		

Prep time: 10 min
Cooking time: 20 min

Ingredients

120g wholemeal flour
1 tsp baking powder
½ tsp cinnamon
a pinch of salt
150g Greek yoghurt
2 eggs
30ml semi-skimmed milk
120g strawberries, chopped into small chunks (plus more to serve)
½ tsp olive oil, for frying
honey and almond butter, to serve

Method

1. Add the wholemeal flour, baking powder, cinnamon and salt to a large bowl and mix.

2. In a separate bowl, mix the Greek yoghurt, eggs and milk together with a fork.

3. Add the wet mixture to the dry mixture and combine to make a soft, thick batter. Add the strawberries and gently mix until evenly dispersed.

4. Use a tablespoon to dollop a quarter of the batter into a non-stick, lightly oiled frying pan. Cook for 2–3 minutes, flip and cook for another 2–3 minutes until golden brown on both sides. Repeat with the rest of the batter.

5. Serve with fresh strawberries, honey and almond butter drizzled on top.

BLUEBERRY AND ALMOND BUTTER PROTEIN PORRIDGE

Serves:	2	Protein (g):	17
Serving:	331g	Fat (g):	11
Calories (kcal):	355	Fibre (g):	5.8
Carbs (g):	43		

Prep time: 5 min
Cooking time: 10 min

Ingredients

100g oats
300ml unsweetened almond milk
100g blueberries (plus more to serve)
2 tsp honey
2 tsp almond butter (plus more to serve)
4 egg whites

Method

1. Add oats, almond milk, blueberries, honey and almond butter to a small pot and bring to the boil. Reduce heat and simmer for 5–6 minutes.

2. Whisk the egg whites in a bowl with a fork until light and fluffy. Take the porridge mixture off the heat and slowly fold in the egg whites. Put back on the heat for another 1–2 minutes until cooked.

3. Serve with more blueberries and almond butter drizzled on top.

PEAR BAKED OATS

Serves:	2	Protein (g):	9.3
Serving:	340g	Fat (g):	6.6
Calories (kcal):	329	Fibre (g):	7.4
Carbs (g):	55		

Prep time: 10 min

Cooking time: 30 min

Ingredients

½ tsp olive oil

2 pears

80g oats

1 tsp cinnamon

a pinch of salt

250ml semi-skimmed milk

1 tbsp maple syrup

1 tsp vanilla extract

Greek yoghurt and honey, to serve

Method

1. Preheat oven to 200°C/180°C Fan/Gas Mark 6.

2. Lightly coat a baking dish with a little oil.

3. Chop 1½ pears into small chunks and slice the remaining ½ for later.

4. Mix the oats, cinnamon and salt together in a large bowl. Add the milk, maple syrup and vanilla extract and mix well.

5. Transfer the mixture to your greased baking dish, top with sliced pear and bake for 25–30 minutes.

6. Serve with Greek yoghurt and a drizzle of honey.

SIMPLE HOMEMADE GRANOLA

Serves:	6	Protein (g):	9.5
Serving:	66g	Fat (g):	18
Calories (kcal):	315	Fibre (g):	3.4
Carbs (g):	28		

Prep time: 10 min

Cooking time: 30 min

Ingredients

180g oats

100g mixed nuts, slightly crushed

40g mixed seeds

2 tbsp coconut oil, melted

50ml maple syrup

Greek yoghurt and fresh berries, to serve

Method

1. Preheat your oven to 200°C/180°C Fan/Gas Mark 6 and line a baking tray with parchment paper.

2. Mix the oats, mixed nuts and seeds together in a large bowl.

3. Add the coconut oil and maple syrup to the dry ingredients. Combine well and spread evenly onto the lined baking tray.

4. Bake for 20–30 minutes. Allow to cool.

5. Serve with Greek yoghurt and fresh berries. Your granola can also be stored in an airtight container for later.

SPICED SCRAMBLED EGGS WITH SMOKED SALMON AND ASPARAGUS

Serves:	2	Protein (g):	35
Serving:	290g	Fat (g):	18
Calories (kcal):	441	Fibre (g):	6.2
Carbs (g):	31		

Prep time: 10 min

Cooking time: 10 min

Ingredients

4 eggs

½ tsp chilli powder (plus more to serve)

½ tsp olive oil, for frying

100g asparagus, ends removed

100g smoked salmon

4 slices of wholemeal bread, toasted

salt and freshly ground black pepper

Method

1. Whisk the eggs and chilli powder together. Pour into a non-stick, lightly oiled frying pan and cook over a medium heat for 3–5 minutes, stirring continuously until cooked.

2. Bring a pot of water to the boil, reduce the heat and cook the asparagus for 3–5 minutes until cooked through, with a bit of bite.

3. Divide the asparagus and smoked salmon between two slices of wholemeal toast. Add the spiced scrambled eggs and serve with a pinch of chilli powder, salt and pepper.

SHAKSHUKA

Serves:	2	Protein (g):	22
Serving:	601g	Fat (g):	16
Calories (kcal):	371	Fibre (g):	8.4
Carbs (g):	27		

Prep time: 15 min
Cooking time: 25 min

Ingredients

1 tsp olive oil
1 medium onion, finely chopped
1 green pepper, deseeded and sliced
1 red pepper, deseeded and sliced
1 clove of garlic, crushed
½ tsp cumin seed
½ tsp paprika
½ tsp chilli powder
1 tbsp tomato purée
400g tinned tomatoes
1 tsp sugar
handful of fresh parsley, chopped (plus more to serve)
4 eggs
feta cheese, to serve
salt and freshly ground black pepper

Method

1. Heat oil in frying pan over a medium heat. Add the onion, peppers and garlic and fry until just softened.

2. Add the cumin seeds, paprika and chilli powder along with your tomato purée and fry for 1 minute before adding the tinned tomatoes and sugar. Lower the heat and simmer for 8–10 minutes until thickened slightly. The aim is to get the consistency right – add some water if it's too thick, or continue cooking if too thin.

3. When the consistency is right, stir in the parsley. Make 4 wells in the sauce and crack an egg into each. Cook for 3–5 minutes until the eggs are cooked.

4. Crumble feta cheese and extra parsley over the top. Serve with toasted bread of your choice.

SWEETCORN FRITTERS WITH FRIED EGG AND HOMEMADE SALSA

Serves:	2	Protein (g):	24
Serving:	508g	Fat (g):	19
Calories (kcal):	508	Fibre (g):	7
Carbs (g):	54		

Prep time: 15 min

Cooking time: 5 min

Ingredients

1 beef tomato, peeled and finely chopped

1 small red onion, finely chopped

small handful of fresh coriander, chopped

juice of half a lime

80g plain flour

1 tsp baking powder

4 eggs

40ml milk

200g tinned sweetcorn, drained

2 spring onions, chopped

½ tsp olive oil, for frying

Method

1. To make the salsa, mix the tomato, onion, coriander and lime juice together in a small bowl.

2. In a large bowl, mix the plain flour and baking powder together. Add 2 out of the 4 eggs along with the milk, and whisk to form a smooth batter. Add a dash more milk if needed.

3. Fold in the sweetcorn and spring onions until combined.

4. Use a tablespoon to transfer the batter into a non-stick, lightly oiled frying pan to make 4 fritters. Cook on a medium-high heat for 1–2 minutes, flip and cook for a further 1–2 minutes until golden brown on both sides. Set aside.

5. Using the same lightly oiled pan, fry the remaining 2 eggs until cooked to your preference.

6. Serve the sweetcorn fritters with fried egg and salsa on top.

RED PEPPER & FETA PROTEIN MUFFINS

Serves:	6	Protein (g):	11
Serving:	141g	Fat (g):	8.4
Calories (kcal):	140	Fibre (g):	1.4
Carbs (g):	4.2		

Prep time: 15 min
Cooking time: 15 min

Ingredients

½ tsp olive oil
1 onion, finely chopped
1 red pepper, deseeded and chopped
handful of spinach, finely chopped
8 eggs
40g feta cheese

Method

1. Preheat oven to 200°C/180°C Fan/Gas Mark 6. Grease a 12-cup muffin tin with oil.

2. In a medium-sized bowl, mix the onion, pepper and spinach together. Spoon the mixture evenly into each cup of the muffin tin.

3. Whisk the eggs together. Pour the mixture evenly into each cup until almost full and crumble the feta cheese on top.

4. Bake for 12–15 minutes and serve. Your muffins can also be stored in an airtight container for later.

Lunch

A good rule for lunch is to make sure that you have a high-quality protein source and then build the meal around it. In these recipes I've used mackerel, chicken and salmon as the base for the meals, and then other ingredients are added for taste and to make it more nutritionally balanced. In two meals – the veggie chilli stuffed sweet potatoes and butternut squash soup – you'll see that the protein is slightly lower, which means you'd choose a higher protein breakfast and dinner to balance that out. These two recipes are great options if you're looking to increase your vegetable intake or adopt a more plant-based approach to your diet.

MEDITERRANEAN CHOPPED SALAD WITH MACKEREL AND CUCUMBER

Serves:	2	Protein (g):	19
Serving:	424g	Fat (g):	19
Calories (kcal):	303	Fibre (g):	5.3
Carbs (g):	11		

Prep time: 10 min

Cooking time: 12 min

Ingredients

2 mackerel fillets

150g lettuce, chopped

1 beef tomato, chopped

½ cucumber, chopped

1 red pepper, deseeded and chopped

handful of fresh parsley, chopped

juice of half a lemon

handful of mixed seeds

salt and freshly ground black pepper

Method

1. Preheat oven to 180°C/160°C Fan/Gas Mark 4. Line a baking tray with parchment paper.

2. Place mackerel fillets in the baking tray, season with salt and pepper and bake for 10–12 minutes until cooked through. Use a fork to loosen the fillets into flakes.

3. In a large bowl, mix together the lettuce, tomato, cucumber, pepper, parsley and lemon juice.

4. Divide the salad mix between two bowls, and add the flaked mackerel and mixed seeds on top.

ZINGY CHICKEN SALAD AND WHOLEWHEAT PITTA BREAD

Serves:	2	Protein (g):	40
Serving:	345g	Fat (g):	5.1
Calories (kcal):	398	Fibre (g):	5.6
Carbs (g):	45		

Prep time: 15 min
Cooking time: 8 min

Ingredients

2 chicken breasts, diced into small chunks

2 cloves of garlic, crushed

juice of ½ a lemon

1 celery stick, chopped

½ red onion, finely chopped

60g seedless grapes, halved

30g Greek yoghurt

1 tsp olive oil, for frying

2 wholemeal pitta breads, toasted

40g lettuce, chopped

salt and freshly ground black pepper

Method

1. Add the chicken, garlic and lemon juice to a bowl and mix well. Season with salt and pepper and set aside for 10 minutes.

2. Mix the celery, red onion, grapes and Greek yoghurt together in a large bowl.

3. Add the marinated chicken to a non-stick, lightly oiled frying pan and cook over a medium heat for 6–8 minutes until completely cooked through but still moist.

4. Fill the toasted pitta breads with the warm chicken, salad mix and lettuce and serve.

SALMON KEBABS WITH GIANT COUSCOUS AND LIME SWEET CHILLI SAUCE

Serves:	2	Protein (g):	39
Serving:	539g	Fat (g):	21
Calories (kcal):	577	Fibre (g):	6
Carbs (g):	51		

Prep time: 15 min
Cooking time: 8 min

Ingredients

4 tbsp sweet chilli sauce
juice of 1 lime (plus 2 wedges to serve)
2 skinless salmon fillets, diced into chunks
80g giant couscous

160ml water

1 yellow pepper, deseeded and chopped

½ red onion, chopped

1 beef tomato, chopped

small handful fresh mint, chopped

1 tsp olive oil, for frying

Method

1. Mix the sweet chilli sauce and lime juice together in a bowl. Skewer the salmon fillets, cover with the sauce and set aside to marinate for 15–20 minutes.

2. Add the giant couscous and water to a saucepan. Bring to the boil over a medium heat, then reduce heat and simmer for 6–8 minutes until cooked, before setting aside to cool.

3. Once cooled, add to a large bowl with the pepper, red onion, tomato and mint. Mix together.

4. Add the salmon skewers to a non-stick, lightly oiled frying pan and cook over a medium heat for 6–8 minutes until completely cooked through. Turn the skewers every few minutes to avoid burning.

5. Divide the couscous salad mix between two plates. Place the salmon skewers on top and drizzle any leftover sauce over the top.

6. Serve with a wedge of lime on the side.

SLOW COOKER SPICY CHICKEN SOUP

Serves:	6	Protein (g):	12
Serving:	350g	Fat (g):	0.9
Calories (kcal):	91	Fibre (g):	2.3
Carbs (g):	7.1		

Prep time: 15 min

Cooking time: 6 hrs

Ingredients

2 chicken breasts

3 garlic cloves, crushed

1 onion, chopped

2 celery sticks, chopped

2 carrots, finely diced

1 red chilli, deseeded and finely sliced

400g tinned tomatoes

1l water

1 chicken stock cube

1 tsp chilli powder

1 tsp ground cumin

1 tsp turmeric

salt and freshly ground black pepper

fresh parsley, to garnish

Method

1. Add all the ingredients to your slow cooker and leave to cook for 6 hours on a low-medium heat.

2. After 6 hours, remove the chicken breasts, shred using two forks and return to the slow cooker.

3. Season with more salt and pepper if needed, and garnish with fresh parsley.

4. Serve with your bread of choice.

BUTTERNUT SQUASH SOUP

Serves:	4	Protein (g):	2.7
Serving:	429g	Fat (g):	8.5
Calories (kcal):	171	Fibre (g):	5.6
Carbs (g):	18		

Prep time: 15 min
Cooking time: 70 min

Ingredients

1 butternut squash, deseeded and chopped into cubes
2 carrots, chopped
2 onions, chopped
2 tbsp olive oil, for frying
1 red pepper, deseeded and chopped
1 vegetable stock cube
700ml water
salt and freshly ground black pepper
sour cream and mixed seeds, to garnish

Method

1. Preheat oven to 200°C/180°C Fan/Gas Mark 6.

2. Place butternut squash and carrots onto a baking tray and cook for 30–40 minutes until soft.

3. Add the onions to a non-stick, oiled large saucepan and cook over a medium heat for 4–5 minutes until soft.

4. When the butternut squash and carrots are cooked, add to the saucepan along with the chopped pepper, stock cube, water, salt and pepper. Bring to the boil, then reduce the heat and simmer for 30 mins.

5. Remove from the heat and allow your soup to cool before blending in a food processor or blender. If needed, add more water to get your desired consistency.

6. Re-heat in a saucepan over a low-medium heat.

7. Serve with sour cream and mixed seeds on top, along with your bread of choice.

CHICKEN AND ALMOND TRAYBAKE

Serves:	2	Protein (g):	53
Serving:	499g	Fat (g):	19
Calories (kcal):	531	Fibre (g):	8.3
Carbs (g):	33		

Prep time: 10 min

Cooking time: 40 min

Ingredients

300g of boneless and skinless chicken thigh

1 onion, roughly chopped

300g potatoes, chopped

1 red pepper, deseeded and chopped

1 garlic clove, crushed

1 tsp ground cumin

1 tsp smoked paprika

2 tbsp olive oil

juice of ½ an orange

30g almonds, chopped

chopped parsley, to serve

Method

1. Preheat oven to 200°C/180°C Fan/Gas Mark 6.

2. Add the chicken, onion, potatoes and pepper to a baking tray.

3. In a small bowl, mix together the garlic, cumin, paprika, olive oil and orange juice. Pour over the ingredients in the baking

tray and mix until evenly coated.

4. Place in the oven and cook for 30 minutes. Sprinkle the chopped almonds on top and cook for a further 10 minutes until the chicken is cooked through.

5. Garnish with chopped parsley and serve.

VEGGIE CHILLI STUFFED SWEET POTATOES

Serves:	4	Protein (g):	9.7
Serving:	365g	Fat (g):	9.6
Calories (kcal):	402	Fibre (g):	14
Carbs (g):	62		

Prep time: 15 min
Cooking time: 50 min

Ingredients

4 sweet potatoes
1 red onion, finely chopped
1 garlic clove, crushed
1 tsp olive oil, for frying
400g tinned black beans, drained
100g sweetcorn
100g plum tomatoes, chopped
1 tsp smoked paprika
½ tsp chilli flakes
1 avocado, chopped
juice of 1 lime

salt and freshly ground black pepper
sour cream and coriander, to serve

Method

1. Preheat oven to 200°C/180°C Fan/Gas Mark 6. Line a baking tray with parchment paper.

2. Using a fork, make some holes in each of the sweet potatoes. Place on the baking tray and cook for 40–50 minutes until cooked all the way through.

3. To make the chilli, add the red onion and garlic to a non-stick, lightly oiled frying pan and cook over a medium heat for 4–5 minutes until soft.

4. Add the black beans, sweetcorn, plum tomatoes, smoked paprika and chilli flakes and cook for a further 4–5 minutes until heated through.

5. Mix the avocado and lime juice in a small bowl. Season with salt and pepper.

6. Cut the sweet potatoes in half and pile the chilli and avocado on top. Serve with a dollop of sour cream and coriander on top.

Snacks

There's no real hard and fast rule when it comes to snacks. You could just as easily choose a handful of almonds or a piece of fruit, but if you're looking to broaden your horizon beyond those basic examples, then try out some of these. The energy shake is a particular favourite of mine as it's quick, easy and great for on-the-go. The cashew and raisin oat bars, on the other hand, take about 45 minutes – perfect for a spot of Sunday afternoon batch cooking.

ENERGY SHAKE

Serves:	1	Protein (g):	14
Serving:	305g	Fat (g):	14
Calories (kcal):	307	Fibre (g):	2.9
Carbs (g):	30		

Prep time: 5 min

Ingredients

1 frozen banana

100ml unsweetened almond milk

60g Greek yoghurt

handful of spinach

1 tbsp peanut butter

1 tsp honey

Method

1. Combine all the ingredients using a blender – add more almond milk for a thinner consistency.

CHICKEN SKEWERS WITH GREEK YOGHURT DIP

Serves:	2	Protein (g):	40
Serving:	390g	Fat (g):	13
Calories (kcal):	335	Fibre (g):	2.7
Carbs (g):	13		

Prep time: 30 min

Cooking time: 8 min

Ingredients

1 tbsp olive oil

juice of 1 lemon

1 garlic clove, crushed

2 chicken breasts, diced into chunks

1 red onion, chopped

1 yellow pepper, deseeded and chopped

150g Greek yoghurt

1 tsp dried parsley

1 tsp dried basil

½ tsp garlic powder

½ tsp onion powder

salt and freshly ground black pepper

Method

1. Mix the olive oil, lemon juice and garlic in a bowl. Add the diced chicken breasts, season with salt and pepper and set aside to marinate for 15–20 minutes.

2. Skewer the chicken, red onion and pepper. Add the remaining marinade to a non-stick frying pan, add the skewers and cook over a medium heat for 6–8 minutes, until completely cooked through but still moist.

3. To make the dip, mix the Greek yoghurt, parsley, basil, garlic powder and onion powder in a bowl and serve alongside the hot chicken skewers.

AVOCADO TOAST WITH COTTAGE CHEESE

Serves:	2	Protein (g):	10
Serving:	290g	Fat (g):	12
Calories (kcal):	294	Fibre (g):	7.4
Carbs (g):	31		

Prep time: 10 min

Ingredients

4 slices wholemeal sourdough bread, toasted
4 tbsp cottage cheese
1 ripe avocado, sliced
2 beef tomato, sliced
salt and freshly ground black pepper
chilli flakes, optional

Method

1. Spread the cottage cheese on top of the toasted sourdough bread.

2. Place the avocado and tomato slices on top, and season with salt and pepper.

3. Sprinkle chilli flakes on top and serve.

COCONUT BERRY SMOOTHIE

Serves:	1	Protein (g):	6.9
Serving:	347g	Fat (g):	4.9
Calories (kcal):	227	Fibre (g):	5.1
Carbs (g):	35		

Prep time: 5 min

Ingredients

1 frozen banana

60g strawberries

30g raspberries

50g Greek yoghurt

100ml unsweetened coconut milk

1 tsp honey

Method

1. Combine all the ingredients using a blender – add more coconut milk for a thinner consistency.

CASHEW AND RAISIN OAT BARS

Serves:	8	Protein (g):	7.2
Serving:	76g	Fat (g):	8.2
Calories (kcal):	218	Fibre (g):	2.7
Carbs (g):	28		

Prep time: 15 min

Cooking time: 35 min

Ingredients

180g oats

40g sugar

1½ tsp baking powder

pinch of salt

2 eggs

120ml semi-skimmed milk

1 tsp vanilla extract

60g raisins

80g cashews, roughly chopped

Method

1. Preheat oven to 200°C/180°C Fan/Gas Mark 6. Line a baking tin with parchment paper.

2. In a large bowl, mix the oats, sugar, baking powder and salt together.

3. In a smaller bowl, whisk the eggs, milk and vanilla extract together.

4. Add the wet ingredients into the dry ingredients and mix well. Fold in the raisins and cashew nuts.

5. Spread the combined mixture into the prepared baking tin and flatten with the back of a spoon.

6. Bake for 30–35 minutes until golden brown.

7. Allow to cool on a wire rack and then cut into 8 bars. These can be stored in an airtight container for later.

Dinner

On to my favourite meal of the day! As at lunchtime, try and aim for a high-quality protein source as your meal's base and then add around it. Most of the protein and carbohydrate sources are interchangeable here, too; you could use chicken or turkey instead of pork in the stir-fry, for example, or substitute sweet potatoes for brown rice in the slow cooker chilli con carne. Find what works best for you. Another tip for those short on time is to make extra food at dinner and then use it for lunch the following day.

GARLIC AND HERB ROASTED CHICKEN AND VEGETABLES

Serves:	4	Protein (g):	13
Serving:	457g	Fat (g):	2.3
Calories (kcal):	341	Fibre (g):	7.8
Carbs (g):	64		

Prep time: 15 min

Cooking time: 35 min

Ingredients

4 garlic cloves, crushed

2 tbsp apple cider vinegar

2 tbsp olive oil

2 tsp dried thyme

2 tsp dried rosemary

4 chicken breasts

2 red onions, chopped

2 large sweet potatoes, chopped into cubes

100g brussels sprouts, outer leaves removed and halved

2 green apples, cored and sliced

salt and freshly ground black pepper

Method

1. Preheat oven to 200°C/180°C Fan/Gas Mark 6. Line a baking tray with parchment paper.

2. Mix the garlic, apple cider vinegar, oil, thyme and rosemary together in a large bowl.

3. Add the chicken breasts and coat in the mixture, season with salt and pepper and set aside to marinate.

4. Place the red onion, sweet potato, brussels sprouts and apple on the baking tray. Set the chicken breasts on top and drizzle over any of the remaining marinade.

5. Cook for 30–35 minutes until the chicken is cooked through and the vegetables are golden brown.

PESTO TURKEY NOODLES

Serves:	2	Protein (g):	48
Serving:	294g	Fat (g):	22
Calories (kcal):	561	Fibre (g):	4
Carbs (g):	41		

Prep time: 10 min
Cooking time: 10 min

Ingredients

300g turkey breast steaks, cut into strips
1 tsp olive oil
100g dried whole wheat noodles
50g basil pesto
100g cherry tomatoes
25g grated parmesan cheese (plus more to serve)
salt and freshly ground black pepper
fresh basil, to garnish

Method

1. Add the sliced turkey breast steaks to a non-stick, lightly oiled frying pan over a medium heat and cook for 5–7 minutes until cooked through. Set aside.

2. Add the noodles to a saucepan of boiling water and cook for 6–7 minutes over a medium heat until soft.

3. Add noodles, pesto, cherry tomatoes and parmesan cheese to the frying pan with the turkey and cook over a low heat for 2–3 minutes, stirring until combined and heated through. Season with salt and pepper as needed.

4. Serve with extra parmesan cheese on top and garnish with fresh basil.

SWEET POTATO CHICKEN CURRY WITH QUINOA

Serves:	4	Protein (g):	37
Serving:	524g	Fat (g):	25
Calories (kcal):	578	Fibre (g):	8.5
Carbs (g):	47		

Prep time: 15 min

Cooking time: 45 min

Ingredients

200g sweet potato, chopped into cubes

400ml coconut milk

1 onion, chopped

2 garlic clove, crushed

1 tsp fresh ginger, grated

1 tbsp olive oil

3 chicken breasts, diced into chunks

1 red pepper, deseeded and chopped

1 yellow pepper, deseeded and chopped

3 tsp curry powder

1 tsp cumin

1 tsp chilli powder

1 tsp dried coriander

200g quinoa

400ml water

salt and freshly ground black pepper

fresh coriander, to garnish

Method

1. Place sweet potato in a saucepan of water over a medium heat. Bring to the boil and cook for 12–14 minutes until soft (the smaller the cubes, the shorter the cooking time).

2. Once cooked and drained, allow to cool slightly before using a blender to blend the sweet potato and coconut milk together.

3. Add the onion, garlic and ginger to a non-stick, lightly oiled frying pan and cook for 4–5 minutes until the onions have softened.

4. Add the chicken and cook for 3–5 minutes until sealed (i.e. the outside of the chicken has turned white). Add the peppers and cook for a further 12–15 minutes. Add a splash of water if things are starting to stick to the pan.

5. Add the curry powder, cumin, chilli powder and dried coriander and cook for 1–2 minutes, before adding the sweet potato and coconut milk mixture.

6. Lower the heat and simmer for 5–7 minutes until the chicken is cooked through and the sauce thickens. Season with salt and pepper as needed.

7. Add your quinoa and water to a saucepan and bring to the boil over a medium heat. Reduce the heat and simmer for 12–15 minutes.

8. Serve the curry in bowls, spooned over the quinoa with fresh coriander on top to garnish.

STEAK WITH BABY POTATOES AND HOMEMADE COLESLAW

Serves:	2	Protein (g):	46
Serving:	451g	Fat (g):	41
Calories (kcal):	668	Fibre (g):	6.2
Carbs (g):	25		

Prep time: 10 min

Cooking time: 15 min

Ingredients

2 sirloin steaks

250g baby potatoes

1 carrot, grated

¼ red cabbage, finely shredded

3 tbsp mayonnaise

1 tbsp apple cider vinegar

1 tsp mustard

salt and freshly ground black pepper

1 tbsp olive oil

Method

1. Remove the steaks from the fridge for 15–20 minutes, to allow them to get to room temperature.

2. Cook the potatoes in a large pot of boiling water for 12–15 minutes over a low-medium heat until tender.

3. To make the coleslaw, mix the carrot, red cabbage, mayonnaise, apple cider vinegar and mustard together in a large bowl. Season with salt and pepper and set aside.

4. Brush both sides of the steak with olive oil and season with salt and pepper. Cook on a hot, non-stick griddle pan for 2–4 minutes on both sides until cooked to your preference. Set aside and allow to rest for 2–4 minutes before serving with potatoes and coleslaw.

ROASTED CURRY SALMON AND BROWN RICE

Serves:	2	Protein (g):	34
Serving:	580g	Fat (g):	25
Calories (kcal):	437	Fibre (g):	6.7
Carbs (g):	14		

Prep time: 10 min
Cooking time: 30 min

Ingredients

1 beef tomato, sliced
2 salmon fillets
1 tbsp olive oil
1 tbsp curry powder
120g brown rice
1 carrot, chopped into small chunks
240ml water

80g frozen peas
salt and freshly ground black pepper
fresh coriander, to garnish

Method

1. Preheat oven to 180°C/160°C Fan/Gas Mark 4. Line a baking tray with parchment paper.

2. Lay the tomatoes on the lined baking tray and place the salmon fillets on top.

3. Mix the olive oil and curry powder together in a small bowl before brushing over the salmon fillets. Cook for 15–20 minutes until the salmon is cooked.

4. Next add your rice, carrot and water to a saucepan and bring to the boil over a medium heat. Reduce the heat and simmer for 20–25 minutes. Add the peas and cook for a further 5 minutes.

5. Divide the rice into two bowls and place the salmon fillets on top. Garnish with fresh coriander and serve.

BAKED FALAFEL BURGERS AND HOMEMADE CHIPS

Serves:	2	Protein (g):	18
Serving:	312g	Fat (g):	15
Calories (kcal):	578	Fibre (g):	11
Carbs (g):	87		

Prep time: 15 min

Cooking time: 50 min

Ingredients

1 large baking potato

1 tbsp olive oil

2 garlic cloves, crushed

handful of fresh parsley, chopped

½ tsp turmeric

juice of 1 lemon

200g tinned chickpeas, drained

20g plain flour

2 brioche buns

salt and freshly ground black pepper

lettuce, tomato and sauce of choice, to serve

Method

1. Preheat oven to 180°C/160°C Fan/Gas Mark 4. Line two baking trays with parchment paper.

2. Chop the potato into chips, toss in olive oil and season with salt and pepper. Place on one of your lined baking trays and cook for 40–50 minutes until golden and crispy.

3. To make the burgers, add the garlic, parsley, turmeric and lemon juice to a food processor and pulse.

4. Add the chickpeas and flour, and pulse until the mixture starts to come together.

5. Split the mixture in two and form into burger shapes. Place these in the fridge for 20 minutes to firm up.

6. When firm, place your burgers on the other lined baking tray and cook for 25–30 minutes, turning halfway through cooking.

7. Toast the brioche buns and build your burgers with lettuce, tomato and a sauce of your choice. Serve alongside the homemade chips.

SLOW COOKER CHILLI CON CARNE WITH BROWN RICE

Serves:	6	Protein (g):	22
Serving:	519g	Fat (g):	15
Calories (kcal):	312	Fibre (g):	7.9
Carbs (g):	17		

Prep time: 20 min

Cooking time: 8 hrs

Ingredients

500g beef, minced

1 tsp olive oil

1 onion, chopped

2 celery sticks, chopped

2 garlic cloves, crushed

1 beef stock cube

200ml warm water

400g tinned kidney beans, drained

400g tinned tomatoes

2 tbsp tomato purée

1 carrot, chopped

1 red pepper, deseeded and chopped

1 tbsp chilli powder

2 tsp smoked paprika

2 tsp cumin

2 tsp turmeric

2 tsp dried coriander

360g brown rice
720ml water
salt and freshly ground black pepper
Greek yoghurt and fresh coriander, to serve

Method

1. Add the minced beef to a non-stick, lightly oiled frying pan and cook for 5–10 minutes until browned. Transfer your meat into the slow cooker.

2. Add the onion, celery and garlic to the frying pan and cook for 4–5 minutes until softened slightly. Transfer to the slow cooker.

3. Dissolve your stock cube in 200ml of warm water.

4. Add the stock and the remaining ingredients – except for the rice – to the slow cooker. Season with salt and pepper and cook on a low heat for 6–8 hours.

5. Add your rice and water to a saucepan and bring to the boil over a medium heat. Reduce the heat and simmer for 25–30 minutes until cooked.

6. Serve the chilli con carne in bowls, spooned over the rice with a dollop of Greek yoghurt and fresh coriander on top.

PORK AND VEGETABLE STIR-FRY

Serves:	2	Protein (g):	37
Serving:	499g	Fat (g):	26
Calories (kcal):	625	Fibre (g):	9.8
Carbs (g):	56		

Prep time: 15 min

Cooking time: 15 min

Ingredients

250g pork loin medallions, diced

2 tbsp soy sauce

2 tsp fish sauce

1 tsp Chinese five spice

1 tsp brown sugar

1 tbsp olive oil

1 onion, chopped

1 garlic clove, crushed

1 tsp fresh ginger, grated

½ red chilli, finely chopped

1 red pepper, deseeded and sliced

150g mangetout

100g pak choi, chopped

100g dried whole wheat noodles

crushed peanuts, to garnish

Method

1. Add the pork, soy sauce, fish sauce, Chinese five sauce and brown sugar to a bowl and mix until the pork is evenly coated.

2. Add the pork and sauce to a non-stick, lightly oiled frying pan over a medium heat and cook for 3–5 minutes until cooked through. Set the pork aside.

3. In the same frying pan, cook the onion, garlic, ginger, chilli and pepper over a medium heat for 4–5 minutes until soft. Add the pork back in along with the mangetout and pak choi, and cook for 2–3 minutes.

4. Add the noodles to a saucepan of boiling water and cook for 6–7 minutes over a medium heat until soft. Drain.

5. Serve the stir-fried pork and vegetables over the cooked noodles. Garnish with crushed peanuts and serve.

Endnotes

1. Evenepoel, C.; Clevers, E.; Deroover, L.; Van Loo, W.; Matthys, C.; Verbeke, K. (2020). 'Accuracy of Nutrient Calculations Using the Consumer-Focused Online App MyFitnessPal: Validation Study.' *Journal of Medical Internet Research*, 22 (10): e18237.

2. Cherry, K. (2020). 'How Cognitive Biases Influence How You Think and Act.' Verywell Mind. https://www.verywellmind.com/what-is-a-cognitive-bias-2794963.

3. Karra, E.; Chandarana, K.; Batterham, R. L. (2009). 'The Role of Peptide YY in Appetite Regulation and Obesity.' *The Journal of Physiology*, 587 (1): 19–25.

4. Levesque, Crystal L. and Ball, Ronald O. 'Protein and Amino Acid Requirements.' Basicmedical Key. https://basicmedicalkey.com/protein-and-amino-acid-requirements/.

5. Coelho do Vale, R.; Pieters, R.; Zeelenberg, M. (2016). 'The Benefits of Behaving Badly on Occasion: Successful Regulation by Planned Hedonic Deviations.' *Journal of Consumer Psychology*, 26 (1): 17–28.

6. Melini, V. and Melini, F. (2019). 'Gluten-Free Diet: Gaps and Needs for a Healthier Diet.' *Nutrients*, 11 (1): 170.

7. Crichton, G. E.; Elias, M. F.; Dore, G. A.; Robbins, M. A. (2012). 'Relation Between Dairy Food Intake and Cognitive Function: The Maine-Syracuse Longitudinal Study.' *International Dairy Journal*, 22 (1): 15–23.

8. Wang, Y. M. and Eys, J. (1981). 'Nutritional Significance of Fructose and Sugar Alcohols.' *Annual Review of Nutrition*, 1 (1): 437–75.

9. Mäkinen, Kauko K. (2016). 'Gastrointestinal Disturbances Associated with the Consumption of Sugar Alcohols with Special Consideration of Xylitol: Scientific Review and Instructions for Dentists and Other Health-Care Professionals.' *International Journal of Dentistry*, 2016: 1–16.

10. Ruiz-Ojeda, F. J.; Plaza-Díaz, J.; Sáez-Lara, M. J.; Gil, A. (2019). 'Effects of Sweeteners on the Gut Microbiota: A Review of Experimental Studies and Clinical Trials.' *Advances in Nutrition*, 10: S31–48.

11. Katan, M. B.; Brouwer, I. A.; Clarke, R.; Geleijnse, J. M; Mensink, R. P. (2010). 'Saturated Fat and Heart Disease.' *The American Journal of Clinical Nutrition*, 92 (2): 459–60.

12. Oteng, Antwi-Boasiako and Kersten, S. (2019). 'Mechanisms of Action of Trans Fatty Acids.' *Advances in Nutrition*, November.

13. Lehnen, T. E.; Ramos da Silva, M.; Camacho, A.; Marcadenti, A.; Machado Lehnen, A. (2015). 'A Review on Effects of Conjugated Linoleic Fatty Acid (CLA) Upon Body Composition and Energetic Metabolism.' *Journal of the International Society of Sports Nutrition*, 12 (1).

14. Azain, M. J.; Hausman, D. B.; Sisk, M. B.; Flatt, W. P.; Jewell, D. E. (2000). 'Dietary Conjugated Linoleic Acid Reduces Rat Adipose Tissue Cell Size rather than Cell Number.' *The Journal of Nutrition*, 130 (6): 1548–54.

15. Schoenfeld, B. J.; Aragon, A. A.; Wilborn, C. D.; Krieger, J. W.; Sonmez, G. T. (2014). 'Body Composition Changes Associated with Fasted versus Non-Fasted Aerobic Exercise.' *Journal of the International Society of Sports Nutrition*, 11 (1).

16. D'Andrea Meira, I.; Taynan Romão, T.; Pires do Prado, H. J.; Krüger, L. T.; Paiva Pires, M. E.; Oliveira da Conceição, P. (2019). 'Ketogenic Diet and Epilepsy: What We Know so Far.' *Frontiers in Neuroscience*, 13 (5).

17. Levine, J. A. (2002). 'Non-Exercise Activity Thermogenesis (NEAT).' *Best Practice & Research Clinical Endocrinology & Metabolism*, 16 (4): 679–702.

18. van Uffelen, J. G. Z.; Wong, J.; Chau, J. Y.; van der Ploeg, H. P.; Riphagen, I.; Gilson, N. D.; Burton, N. W. et al. (2010). 'Ocupational Sitting and Health Risks.' *American Journal of Preventive Medicine*, 39 (4): 379–88.

19. Chen, Y.; Tan, F.; Wei, L.; Li, X.; Lyu, Z.; Feng, X.; Wen, Y. et al. (2018). 'Sleep Duration and the Risk of Cancer: A Systematic Review and Meta-Analysis Including Dose–Response Relationship.' *BMC Cancer*, 18 (1).

20. Fischer, D.; Lombardi, D. A.; Marucci-Wellman, H.; Till Roenneberg, T. (2017). 'Chronotypes in the US – Influence of Age and Sex.' *PLOS ONE*, 12 (6): e0178782.

21. White, D.; de Klerk, S.; Woods, W.; Gondalia, S.; Noonan, C.; Scholey, A. (2016). 'Anti-Stress, Behavioural and Magnetoencephalography Effects of an L-Theanine-Based Nutrient Drink: A Randomised, Double-Blind, Placebo-Controlled, Crossover Trial.' *Nutrients*, 8 (1): 53.

22. Kiecolt-Glaser, J. K.; Habash, D. L.; Fagundes, C. P.; Andridge, R.; Peng, J.; Malarkey, W. B.; Belury, M. A. (2015). 'Daily stressors, past depression, and metabolic responses to high-fat meals: A novel path to obesity.' *Biological Psychiatry Journal*, 77 (7): 653–60.

23. Daubenmier, J.; Kristeller, J.; Hecht, F.M., et al. (2011). 'Mindfulness intervention for stress eating to reduce cortisol and abdominal fat among overweight and obese women: An exploratory randomized controlled study.' *International Journal of Obesity*.

24. Burke, L. E.; Wang, J.; Sevick, M. A. (2011). 'Self-monitoring in weight loss: A systematic review of the literature.' *Journal of the American Dietetic Association*, 111 (1): 92–102.

25. Craft, L. L. and Perna, F. M. (2004). 'The Benefits of Exercise for the Clinically Depressed.' *Primary Care Companion to the Journal of Clinical Psychiatry*, 6 (3): 104–11.

26. Shevchuk, N. A. (2008). 'Adapted Cold Shower as a Potential Treatment for Depression.' *Medical Hypotheses*, 70 (5): 995–1001.

27. Hussain, J. and Cohen, M. (2018). 'Clinical Effects of Regular Dry Sauna Bathing: A Systematic Review.' *Evidence-Based Complementary and Alternative Medicine*, 2018: 1–30.

28. Kouda, K. and Iki, M. (2010). 'Beneficial Effects of Mild Stress (Hormetic Effects): Dietary Restriction and Health.' *Journal of Physiological Anthropology*, 29 (4): 127–32.

Index